COUPLE THERAPY WITH GAY MEN

The Guilford Family Therapy Series

Michael P. Nichols, Series Editor

Recent Volumes

Couple Therapy with Gay Men

DAVID E. GREENAN
GIL TUNNELL

Foreword by Salvador Minuchin

THE GUILFORD PRESS
New York   London

© 2003 The Guilford Press
A Division of Guilford Publications, Inc.
72 Spring Street, New York, NY 10012
www.guilford.com

Printed in the United States of America

This book is printed on acid-free paper.

Last digit is print number: 9   8   7   6   5   4   3   2   1

Library of Congress Cataloging-in-Publication Data

Greenan, David E.
  Couple therapy with gay men / David E. Greenan, Gil Tunnell ; foreword
by Salvador Minuchin.
      p. cm. — (Guilford family therapy series)
Includes bibliographical references and index.
  ISBN 1-57230-808-7 (hbk. : alk. paper)
  1. Gay couples—Mental health. 2. Marital psychotherapy. I. Tunnell,
Gil. II. Title. III. Series.
  RC558 .G745 2003
  616.89′14′086642—dc21

                                                              2002012811

About the Authors

David E. Greenan, EdD, is Executive Director of The Minuchin Center for the Family, where he teaches family therapy and consults to agencies that serve inner-city poor families. He is also a psychologist and family therapist in private practice in New York City.

Gil Tunnell, PhD, is a clinical psychologist in full-time private practice in New York City. He supervises and trains psychiatric residents and psychology interns in family therapy at Beth Israel Medical Center.

Foreword

It is not often that the title of a book promises less than the book contains, but this book is an exception. When I started reading, I expected to find myself on a road I have traveled before, where I would encounter structural family therapy, joining, enactment, unbalancing, and so forth, along with creative variations, perhaps, and ingenious maneuvers. It is, after all, a book about couples, and I thought I knew all the shapes in which couples are found. Fortunately, I was wrong. The reader will certainly find discussions of therapeutic techniques, but if you allow yourself to move beyond the techniques, as I did, you may find yourself in uncomfortable, though interesting, territory.

I know that my knowledge of gender was shaped by my Argentine culture. Not the "Marlboro Man" but its equivalent in the Argentine gaucho: strong, aggressive but respectful, able to overcome fear without showing emotion, and so on. It is one of the traditional versions by which we identify maleness. But as an enlightened professional, I knew I had overcome the 19th-century version of gender in favor of a more nuanced view that is respectful of diversity. I was taken aback, therefore, when I read about the development of identity in a gay male: the pain, the isolation, the secrecy, the trying to pass, the incorporation of a demeaned self. I recognized the puzzlement and the "why" questions that I have seen in many members of persecuted minorities, including my own experience as a Jew.

The book made me question my equanimity about gender, and made me think about my own homophobia—not in relationships with personal gay friends, I hope, but through an insidious bias based on ignorance and on selective inattention. At that level, we need to thank the authors for their guidance in understanding ourselves. But they go beyond that, connecting the issues of identity formation with the characteristics and problems that affect gay men when they enter into couplehood. What is the road map for intimacy among males? Can members of a gay couple allow themselves to be vulnerable with their partners? What is the therapeutic process that expands the experience of a gay couple beyond the accepted norms of the dominant culture for intimacy? In order to elucidate these questions, the book presents case excerpts that are written in a form that invites you into the office, where you can observe the respectful way in which therapy moves from support to challenge and to the expansion and incorporation of complexity. At this level, Greenan and Tunnell deliver what they have promised: a guide for therapy with gay couples that is clear, practical, and useful. The combination of levels makes the reading of this book a rewarding and complex journey.

SALVADOR MINUCHIN, MD

Preface

Men struggle with other men in our desire to be gentle, supportive, and collaborative with one another. In addition, gay men struggle with the stereotype that we are incapable of sustaining intimate coupled relationships. This book is a basic introduction for therapists new to working with couples and who are specifically interested in learning about the interpersonal dynamics that all men share in negotiating spousal relationships as well as the characteristics that are unique to gay male couples. We also hope that the nonprofessional gay or straight reader, in or desirous of a couple relationship, will find the material inspiring and perhaps transformational.

THE CHAINS OF CULTURE

Writing a book on how we think about gay male acculturation and development, and how our thinking influences the ways we intervene with male couples, presented us with a dilemma. We knew from our personal and clinical experience that the ways in which men are acculturated have specific implications for gay male development and help to organize a therapist's interventions as well. Our dilemma was how to be mindful of these contextual issues of gender acculturation and gay identity development and still remain open to intervening with clients. It's easy for therapists to be held hostage and remain blind to the possibilities for growth through inadvertent absorption of certain cultural stereotypes about males and our capacity for intimate relationships.

Although the civil rights and the feminist movements have challenged and expanded the ways in which we define ourselves, stereotypes continue to organize the roles of men and women. The "Marlboro Man" syndrome is alive and well in American culture. "Boys don't cry" and "Play to win" are attitudes that permeate our cultural conditioning as we grow into men. Many men whom we see in our clinical practices, regardless of their sexual orientation, are caught in rigid roles that reward aggressiveness and competitiveness. These narrow male role definitions discourage us from accessing our more affiliative, collaborative selves. These rigid roles can be particularly challenging for gay men attempting to build and maintain intimate same-sex relationships.

Gay men not only struggle with what it means to be a man due to traditional socialization as children but, equally significantly, they struggle with what it means to be an isolated and shamed minority. Despite the gay rights movement that dates back to the Stonewall Rebellion in 1969, discrimination against lesbian and gay people continues to be legal in many areas of our country, and only the state of Vermont gives equal civil rights to same-sex unions. The lack of laws giving legal recognition to same-sex unions encourages discrimination and contributes to the instability of same-sex relationships.

The earliest messages internalized by most gay children are that we are inferior to our straight peers. Many of these negative messages come from male peers presumably fearful of their own same-sex feelings and society's taboo against such feelings. If you by chance overhear a group of adolescents hanging out together, the worst label that they can attribute to a male peer (and one that society still tolerates) is "faggot." Fathers, having grown up during less tolerant times, frequently shame their sons for being queer. Childhood and adolescence can be a particularly treacherous journey for gay youth. Gay boys often grow up mistrustful of other males and construct a false self in order to be safe and pass as straight. This learned mistrust of males has profound implications for adult gay male couples that we therapists see in our practices daily.

We have written this book to help therapists, both straight and gay, understand how to work with couples in general, and male couples specifically, and to understand how our thinking informs our clinical interventions. In addition to the scarcity of literature about how to work with male couples, a second impetus for writing this book was that we realized how our knowledge of the cultural conditioning that organizes the interactions of men and male couples might serve to immobilize us.

From our own experience, we know that intimate awareness of how men are acculturated and of how gay identity is developed have great potential for tying a therapist up in knots. All couples, gay and straight, present with complementary roles, constructed and sustained by their relationships and the systems that they interact with. The therapist, to facilitate change, must feel free to challenge the limited way a couple interacts with each other.

The additional knowledge of what it's like to grow up gay in a culture that devalues homosexuality and same-sex relationships can have the unintended consequence of paralyzing a therapist. The information in this volume about gay men's development is intended to provide therapists with the context to normalize the behaviors of male couples and to encourage therapists to push their clients to activate inherent but previously dormant resources. We intend for the historical and psychological material presented in Chapters 1 and 2 to serve as a reference point for the therapist to undertake appropriate interventions with gay couples.

The book is written to help clinicians give themselves permission to push for change in male couples. All couples present for treatment during crisis periods in their developmental life cycles, usually caught in inflexible roles occurring predictably in their lives together. A therapist's task is to help the couple identify these predictable patterns, clarify what complementary behaviors make up and maintain their patterns, and create an atmosphere that encourages a couple to expand their repertoire—to experiment with new ways of relating.

Gay couples frequently come for therapy hopeless about the possibility of their maintaining a stable long-term relationship. Gay men whom we see in our clinical practices often feel isolated, marginalized, and bereft of positive role models who support their desire to be in a coupled relationship. In this cultural context men, straight and gay, need therapists who are supportive of and comfortable with providing the necessary therapeutic conditions that encourage man-to-man intimacy. Gay couples additionally need therapists who are willing to challenge destructive behaviors that undermine their chances for survival.

PLAN OF THE BOOK

In Chapters 1 and 2 we give a detailed overview of the early socialization experiences of gay males—how they grow up in ways both similar to and different from straight males as they encounter the culture's rules on "gender-appropriate" behavior—and the stages most gay men go through in adapting to their homosexuality. We apply Bowen's concept of differentiation and Bowlby's theory of attachment and separation to a gay man's individual development to understand the origins of the all-too-common experience of feeling like an undesirable alien in his own country. We examine how these early experiences—rooted in emotional isolation from primary attachment figures, thus rarely enabling a gay man to have an authentic emotional connection with another person who knows and respects his core self—may affect his subsequent ability to form and maintain an intimate coupled relationship with another man. We conclude that, for many men, the early experience of discovering one's homosexuality constitutes a trauma, primarily because the absence of family and social supports forces one to deal with the discovery alone. Confronted with society's heterosexism, homophobia, and strong rules on male gender acculturation, many gay men turn their shame-based aloneness into an overreliance on cultivating personal autonomy and independence, and they may later experience greater difficulty in making deep emotional connections with other men.

Chapter 3 introduces the reader to our basic way of working with a couple through what we describe as a dyadic circular system, the therapeutic model that underlies all of our clinical interventions. Our model is based on Salvador Minuchin's (1974; Minuchin & Fishman, 1981) structural family therapy, a three-stage model for working with families and couples that distinguishes stages based on (1) *joining*, (2) *enactment*, and (3) *unbalancing*. Minuchin's theory of families and family therapy is a health-driven, nonpathologizing treatment model that is particularly appropriate for working with marginalized populations such as gay men because of the potential for the therapy to be a *corrective* experience. Our interventions are buttressed by our strong personal belief that family systems carry within them unrecognized potential and dormant resources. The therapist's task is to help the couple discover these untapped resources.

The three-stage model is intended as a guide so that a therapist does not become overwhelmed by the plethora of details that all couples present with in treatment. Although in application the model is not linear and the experienced family therapist is continually intervening at multiple levels, for a therapist new to working with couples we recommend implementing the three stages sequentially.

In the clinical cases we present, we specifically focus on the here-and-now interactional patterns of a couple's behavioral system and challenge the individuals, also in the here-and-now setting of treatment, to expand their repertoire of behaviors. We encourage a therapist to construct interactional behavior maps of the possible complementary roles a couple has constructed (i.e., distancer and pursuer) as a guide in unbalancing the couple's cycles of destructive behavior. For instance, many gay couples struggle with issues of monogamy. While we don't take a definitive stance for any couple, male couples often desire to open a relationship to avoid conflict over needs that are not being met in their primary relationship.

In the middle and late stages of treatment, the therapist acts as a facilitator in motivating the couple to break up any long-standing destabilizing behavioral patterns. We encourage experimentation with new behaviors in the therapeutic sessions in the belief that a couple is far more complex and resourceful than its initial presentation of itself. To illustrate the generic model and the types of relationship issues that many men struggle with, in Chapter 3 we present the treatment of a heterosexual couple and begin to compare and contrast how our clinical work differs when working specifically with gay male couples.

Mastering this generic three-stage model of family therapy, however, isn't sufficient to work successfully with gay male couples. Each stage of the model requires modification when applied to gay male couples. That is, the technical aspects of joining, enactment, and unbalancing are the treatment map for working with both straight and gay couples. What the therapist pays attention to as he joins, stages enactments, and unbalances the male couple's system, however, is informed by the therapist's understanding of the unique developmental and socialization experiences of gay men. In Chapters 4, 5, and 6 we discuss and illustrate both what is the same and what is different in each stage of therapy when working with gay male couples. For example, male couples, often inclined to avoid conflict, will sometimes threaten to end their relationship when they experience differences. The therapist should make clear that this new stage in their relationship is normal and should simultaneously help the men to accept their differences and begin to accommodate them. Genuine accommodation to other males—rather than submission or dominance—may be a novel experience for a gay man. Grown men may need to learn for the first time that it's OK to take turns and let your partner drive the car, or to ask for help when you're lost.

Throughout, we continually examine how heterosexism, gender

acculturation, homophobia, and gay identity formation emerge in the
therapy sessions, and how gay men and their therapists experience how
these forces are impacting the couple and reckon with them. While our
interventions are designed to create greater flexibility and new behaviors in which the couple can relate with greater satisfaction, we also
know that the interventions are a healing experience for each individual's earlier negative experiences related to coming out and/or gender acculturation. In delineating how to support male couples, we provide a
therapist with information enabling one to differentiate between normal
and acting-out behaviors among gay men.

Using our model, Chapter 7 presents a detailed case study of a male
couple faced with AIDS. As the treatment ends, the couple has evolved
and developed a loving relationship to which many couples, straight or
gay, might aspire. This particular treatment, which occurred almost 10
years ago, led to our current therapeutic emphasis on the necessity of
creating opportunities for gay men in coupled relationships to be more
affiliative and less combative. In Chapter 8 we summarize our conclu-
sions and discuss possibilities for such future treatments as multiple
couple groups that might better address the long-term needs of male
couples struggling for visibility and social legitimacy.

One of the joys in working with gay male couples is that, once they
identify and fully appreciate how their behavior is so constrained and
organized by cultural conditioning, they begin to think and act more
creatively with each other. Both a couple and a therapist can experience
a heightened freedom to be more spontaneous and expressive. Iron-
ically, though gay couples in principle have the creative freedom to
write wholly unconventional scripts for their relationships, in practice
many couples and family therapists end up being unduly constrained by
cultural chains.

For therapists who are gay, it is all too easy to become caught up in
the myriad details that may resonate with one's own experiences or to
feel drafted into the role of savior of one's tribe. Traumatized by many of
the same experiences as their male clients, gay therapists may mirror
their male clients' fears of closeness. From our own experiences, we
provide suggestions for gay therapists to stay the course to remain helpful to the couple's progress.

For therapists who are straight, the book offers information necessary
to work with male couples so as not be overinfluenced by stereotypes
(e.g., that gay men are promiscuous and unable to sustain an intimate
relationship) we all are at risk of internalizing regardless of our sexual

orientation or claims of objectivity. A straight therapist can often feel that she is walking on eggshells in an effort not to come across as homophobic. This volume, in presenting gay men's developmental experiences as normal, gives a therapist permission to push for change.

The struggles of gay couples to conform to male gender stereotypes such as the Marlboro Man and to avoid reexperiencing shameful feelings and memories from earlier periods when each man first realized he was gay are treatment issues unique to working with male couples. In order for the gay couple's treatment to be effective over the long term, therapists must be knowledgeable about and willing to address underlying belief systems and negative experiences from early childhood as they simultaneously push the couple to experiment with new behaviors conducive to a long-term relationship.

What is unique and often inspiring about family therapy, and our model for working with male couples, is that the insight into where the couple is stuck and the experimentation with new, potentially more fulfilling behaviors occurs *right in a therapist's office*. Although we think complexly, our interventions are often simple in session as we encourage a couple to experiment with new ways of relating with each other. The treatment is often short-term and dynamic. Yet, we encourage the therapist to spend extra time in joining with and in terminating therapy with male couples because of the couple's experience of mistrust and isolation from the majority culture.

Male acculturation and gay identity formation are the cultural contexts within which gay men develop. These contexts help shape and organize the male couple as they construct their relationship. And, yet, male couples are similar to all couples in that they must struggle to establish an identity separate from other family systems and learn to accommodate to each other's needs in creating a culture that prioritizes their love for each other. If a family therapist, new or experienced, becomes organized exclusively by cultural context, this knowledge can inhibit the therapist from challenging or encouraging a male couple to experiment with new and more satisfying behavioral patterns. This is true for either straight or gay therapists. Gay therapists can easily be held hostage by their own experience as a minority and by automatic identification with a gay couple—just as straight therapists, for fear of appearing homophobic, can feel reticent to challenge behaviors clearly destructive to the stability of the couple. Through our case studies, we demonstrate to therapists how to avoid these potential therapeutic pitfalls.

The joining phase may be lengthened with gay couples as the therapist gains their trust, and the absence of role models may extend the final phase of treatment as the men experiment with new ways of being together. Ultimately, though, a male couple goes through the same process of change as its straight counterpart. A crisis occurs that challenges the men's interpersonal style, treatment creates an intensity of emotion as the couple identifies repetitive complementary behaviors, and the couple experiments with new roles that lead to a redefining of their relationship with more constructive ways of connecting. In that way, male couples are more *like* than different from straight couples in our universal need for connectedness.

Acknowledgments

We dedicate this book to Salvador Minuchin. His inspiration as a teacher, his generosity of spirit, and his sharing of knowledge provided the path for this book to be written.

We thank Mike Nichols, who gave freely of his time and whose clinical and editorial expertise made this book develop from an idea to a reality. We are grateful to our editor, Jim Nageotte of The Guilford Press, who gave us valuable encouragement and feedback, and who kept us on a steady course. We also wish to thank K. K. Waering, Jr. for his insightful editing, Paul Gordon, for his graphic design that captures the spirit of the book, and Anna Nelson, for her attention to details.

We are indebted to the couples and families who trusted us with their relationships. They ultimately have taught us how to work effectively to facilitate connectedness, satisfaction, and greater intimacy in relationships. Specific clinical examples used in this book are from couples we have worked with, but biographical details have been changed to protect their identities.

We want to acknowledge our colleagues at The Minuchin Center for the Family and Linda Carter of NYU/Bellevue Medical Center, where we each received training in family therapy.

Finally, we wish to thank several persons who read parts of the manuscript at various times and offered extremely useful feedback to us: Sloane Shelton, Jennifer Bryan, Bob Sloboda, Diana Fosha, Jenna Osiason, and Jan Buckaloo. We take full responsibility, however, for the final product.

And, last but not least, we wish to thank our men's peer support group, who for the past 7 years has taught us how to be challenging and provocative and still maintain a loving connectedness. Thanks, guys—Bob, Bud, Fred, and Paul.

David Greenan

I wrote this book partly for Noah in the hope that he will grow up in a world more loving and accepting of differences.

To Sr. Patrice Murphy, Kathleen Perry, and Betsy Selman Babinecz, thank you for your work that changed the direction of my life.

Additionally, I would like to thank Tom Sedlock for the insights he has shared with me over the years, Ilene Cohen and Debra Noumair for their willingness to provide clinical mentoring, and my colleagues at The Minuchin Center for their continuing support, especially George Simon, Ema Genijovich, and Wai-Yung Lee.

Finally, I am deeply indebted to Gil Tunnell, my partner in writing, who held me to a high standard of excellence and discipline. Thank you, my friend.

Gil Tunnell

I want to thank my coauthor, David, for inviting me to collaborate with him. Writing together became a productive synthesis of how two different therapists think about gay male couples and practice family therapy. We have beneficially challenged each other and emerged from our professional collaboration with a friendship stronger than ever.

I wish to acknowledge the "family therapy contingent" at Beth Israel Medical Center, my professional home for the past 10 years. I thank the psychology interns and psychiatric residents I have supervised, as well as my fellow family therapy supervisors, past and present: Dorcas Cofer, Fredlee Kaplan, Elena Taurke Joseph, Mabel Quinones, Joe Rosenthal, and Guy Winch. Although he is not a family therapist, special thanks are owed Harold Been, director of the psychiatry residency training program at Beth Israel, for his steadfast support and for challenging me at lunch 2 years ago on exactly why gay men might have special difficulties with intimacy. Chapter 2 is, by and large, my response to his question.

Six master clinicians merit my special gratitude. Diana Fosha gave thoughtful feedback to earlier drafts of my writing and has inspired me with her own scholarship, her intellectual rigor, and her creativity as a therapist. I met Jenna Osiason as a fellow intern at Bellevue Hospital 20 years ago, and she has become a lifelong friend and colleague. She too provided invaluable feedback on earlier drafts, offered support, and, along with Diana taught me a great deal about valuing human connection where the self can be authentic. To Anne Brooks, I owe special thanks for teaching me about closeness/distance regulation in couples. Ron Frederick and Noah Glassman provided me with key insights on male couples and gay identity development. Elena Taurke Joseph demonstrated to me new ways to help men become more emotionally intimate with one another.

I want to thank my family, who began a journey with me many years ago they were reluctant to take. I thank them—my mother, Iberia, and my siblings, Dick and Mary—for not jumping out of the car when the ride got rough. I also want to thank my two "mother surrogates"— my aunt, Elaine Tunnell Harris, who was my own "Auntie Mame" and who died several months before this book could appear in print, and my mother-in-law, Viola Sloboda. Both women have been faithful allies.

Finally, I thank my partner of 20 years, Robert Sloboda. Not only has he been a mainstay of love and constant support to me in everything I do—truly the "wind beneath my wings"—he developed new capacities during the writing of this book as editor and taskmaster. He told me when a paragraph didn't make sense, and he gently nudged me back to the computer on many a Sunday afternoon, saying, "Don't you think you should be writing right now?" I am most grateful to him for a partnership that enables me to be real.

Contents

COUPLE THERAPY WITH GAY MEN

CHAPTER ONE

The Marginalization of Gay Male Couples

Near the final session of a 6-month treatment of a gay male couple, one of the men mentioned offhandedly that their 25th anniversary would occur the following week. Excited for them, the therapist asked how they would celebrate. The men said they had no plans. As 25 years together is an achievement for any couple, and given this couple's recent recommitment as an outcome of the therapy, some sort of ritual celebration seemed in order. The therapist knew Kurt and Rob were not officially "out" to their families, their employers, or neighbors, either as gay individuals or as a male couple. Unofficially, however, both sets of parents seemed to know that Kurt and Rob were more than friends. Over the years, each family of origin had incorporated the son's "special friend" into its extended family, including him in family gatherings and holiday celebrations. When the couple was on the verge of breaking up, Rob's mother sensed something was wrong and expressed sadness that she was not seeing Kurt as often. But never in their 25 years together had either family explicitly referred to the men as "a couple." The therapist also recalled the startled look on the men's faces during the initial consultation when he rather casually referred to them as "a couple."

When the therapist suggested some sort of anniversary party to honor their quarter-century together, Kurt and Rob stared at the therapist as though he were from another planet and quickly dismissed his idea. They did agree that a quiet romantic dinner for just the two of them would be fun, and they began discussing possible restaurants. As the therapist listened, he asked himself why these men were so reticent to celebrate 25 years together. It suddenly occurred to him that these men had met in 1971, only 2 years after the Stonewall Rebellion in Greenwich Village, where the couple had always lived. The riots at the Stonewall Tavern are generally credited with launching the gay rights movement, where for the first time in U.S. history, gay people asserted their civil rights to the dominant culture, ending centuries of secretiveness for homosexuals. Although gay couples certainly existed before 1969, few couples acknowledged their relationships publicly. In fact, the primary focus of the gay rights movement was an emphasis not on forming long-term same-sex relationships but rather asserting one's individuality, in terms of individual civil rights and individual sexual freedom. Thousands of gay individuals came out of the closet over the next decade, but most gay couples remained underground. Aware that Kurt and Rob might have a unique perspective on becoming a male couple during that era, the therapist asked them what it had been like.

Kurt smiled as he recalled the details. He had actually been inside the Stonewall Tavern that summer night in 1969 when the New York City police raided the bar. Kurt described his excitement and fear over the next few days as homosexuals and their supporters defied the police. Periodic raids on clandestine meeting places for homosexuals were common then, but this particular raid turned out to have a very different consequence.

A major thrust of the movement over the next decade was sexual liberation. Sexual activity between men became much more widespread as the gay community emerged from its underground subculture. The community remained centered around sex. What changed was that gay men were no longer subject to arrest when they congregated in their meeting places—bars, private clubs, and bathhouses. Having multiple sex partners became something of a norm in the urban gay male subculture.

Rob and Kurt had, in fact, met in a sex club in 1971 and had immediately liked each other. After a year of seeing each other (Rob reminded the therapist that in those days no one referred to their encounters as "dates"), they moved in together. From the beginning, they chose not to be monogamous. They told each other of their sexual exploits outside the relationship and sometimes cruised together. But their nonmonogamous ways confused a number of potential sex partners, as well as their gay friends, who thought it "weird" either to be in a relationship amid all the sexual freedom or to be pursuing sexual freedom while in a relationship. The confusion over their arrangement mostly reflected the cultural norm that being a couple implied monogamy. As these men got so many questions from others, they stopped mentioning their relationship altogether when cruising others. In addition, they never presented themselves socially as a couple. *For the first 15 years of their 25-year relationship, they did not know even one other gay male couple.* Kurt and Rob had concealed their relationship not only from the mainstream culture but also from the gay subculture, a fact the therapist never fully appreciated until that session, almost at the end of treatment.

A major issue for this couple (as for many other male couples) had been establishing their identity with boundaries that others recognized and that the couple itself could use to differentiate itself as a social unit. Often in gay male relationships monogamy is not a chief means of forming a common boundary (Johnson & Keren, 1996). If monogamy does not serve this function, what does? What does being a couple mean?

Actually, the problem the couple had brought to therapy was that Rob had fallen in love with an outside sex partner. One by-product of the affair was Rob's realization of what had been missing in his relationship with his long-term partner, a common experience during affairs and one that often precipitates a breakup of the primary relationship. For Rob, the missing component was intimacy, both emotional and sexual. When the men began treatment, they had not had sex with each other for the past five years, which they identified as their primary problem. Although the affair had ended, it had catapulted the couple's relationship into a crisis demanding greater clarity from each: exactly what was their relationship to each other?

Rob and Kurt's entire 25-year relationship had been closeted, shrouded in secrecy, and lacking an identity recognized by either their family and straight friends or their gay friends and acquaintances. While other gay couples may create a "family of choice" (Westin, 1991)—composed of gay and straight singles and couples supportive of their relationship, especially when the family of origin is not—this was not the case for Kurt and Rob. Their relationship had been hidden from virtually everyone, despite their loyal and committed bond of 25 years. They had been, in essence, an invisible couple. Without external social support—this "social oxygen," as April Martin has called it (Martin & Tunnell, 1993)—one wonders how the couple had survived at all.

Over the 6 months of couple treatment, Kurt and Rob were helped to appraise their relationship and to decide whether they wanted to stay together. It seemed to the therapist that often they were trying to figure out whether they had ever been, or now wished to be, a couple. What did it mean to be a male couple?[1] Reviewing with the therapist the details of their relationship, they began to realize just how deeply attached they were, how they depended on the other in a crisis, how they shared a household, how their lives were intertwined economically through various real estate ventures, how much they enjoyed each other as companions, and how they had become each other's best friend. Still, were they "a couple"?

Despite a high level of familiarity and ease with each other, the relationship lacked emotional intensity and sexual passion. Yes, they were housemates, buddies, and financial partners, but did all that make them a couple? As the therapy continued, the men acknowledged how rarely they shared with each other the intimate details of their day-to-day experience, and also how they had never learned to resolve conflicts between them. Instead, over the years they had developed increasingly separate parallel lives.

The therapist began to challenge them in session to experiment with new patterns of relating that allowed for greater emotional self-disclosure rather than their customary withdrawal and retreat. As they talked more to each other in session and increasingly out of session, they slowly became more emotionally connected. This increased emotional closeness, as it happened, led to increased sexual intimacy, a consequence not necessarily intended by the therapist and which surprised the men. In timidly revealing to the therapist they had begun having sex again, they commented that sex now seemed more like "making love" than "having sex." Although the couple made an emotional recommitment to each other by the end of treatment, they elected to maintain their nonmonogamous sexual contract.

In retrospect, in his work with these men the therapist had stood witness to their relationship while challenging the men to deepen it, specifically by becoming more emotionally available to each other. More than resolving specific concrete problems, Kurt and Rob had had their couplehood affirmed and legitimized by the therapist, a recognition

---

[1] See Green and Mitchell (2002) for an excellent discussion on the "relational ambiguity" often present in gay couples.

they had failed to receive anywhere else. The lack of social community to validate them as a couple—a source of support most heterosexual couples take for granted—had severely undermined the couple's very existence. They had lacked the conditions to create a boundary as a couple, an essential task in couplehood (Nichols & Minuchin, 1999). Much as the old African proverb relates that it takes a village to raise a child, similarly it takes a community to sustain and nurture a couple.

OSTRACIZED FIRST AS GAY INDIVIDUALS, LATER AS GAY COUPLES

We will describe in Chapter 2 how gay males, when growing up, rarely have a family or community who validates their core being. Gay men generally report having felt isolated, lonely, and secretive during their childhood and adolescence (Savin-Williams, 1998). Gay youth normally cannot depend on their families to be a safe harbor from the homophobic prejudice of the outside world, and usually do not come out to the family until they are somewhat more secure emotionally or financially. In no other discriminated group does prejudice have such an insidious impact on the developmental process of early ego identity formation. Because African American parents, for example, share with the child the same identifying characteristic—skin color—that can become the basis for discrimination and mistreatment in the outside world, many African American parents specifically teach their children how to cope with whatever prejudice they encounter (Boyd-Franklin, 1993; Hardy, 1993). Most African American children experience at least their home as a zone free of prejudice.

In contrast, in a homophobic culture, gay boys typically get no help from their families in developing a gay identity. Parents may well be the first people to discriminate against a gay boy. If he shows fairly typical early signs of being gay by displaying gender-atypical behavior such as playing with dolls or cross-dressing (Bailey & Zucker, 1995), his nervous parents may send him to a mental health professional, who may further stigmatize him with a diagnosis of gender identity disorder and counsel the parents to put him in long pants and teach him to play baseball. Due either to explicit or implicit cultural messages that pathologize homosexual development and privilege instead living a heterosexual life (heterosexism), most gay boys learn to keep their emerging

sexual orientation a secret until they feel secure enough with it themselves to tell their families, often not until adulthood.

Just as gay youth grow up isolated in their own families and receive
little or no support for forming a gay identity, many gay male couples
lack a social community to support their identity as a couple. Despite
recent revolutionary changes in society's tolerance of homosexuality,
same-sex relationships rarely achieve a legitimacy equivalent to that of
opposite-sex ones. Not only does the larger culture discriminate against
them, their immediate families may discriminate against them, even
once the relationship becomes visible and is acknowledged. That is,
even after the family recognizes the male couple, the family almost always continues to hold a heterosexist bias, bestowing on the couple a
marginalized status inferior to that of their married children. While a
heterosexual son's coupled relationship is honored and respected the
minute he and his bride walk down the aisle, it may take years before
the same family legitimizes their gay son's relationship with his male
partner. In the case of Kurt and Rob, not only did they not have the benefit of their own families to buffer them from the antigay prejudice of
others, but also they did not have the support of other gay men. They
had formed their relationship at a time when the gay subculture did not
value or support coupled relationships and had never developed their
own "family of choice."

The almost total invisibility of Kurt and Rob's 25-year relationship
may sound extreme, particularly in 2002 when the mainstream culture
appears at times to be more tolerant of same-sex relationships. Yet, if
two gay men formed their coupled relationship prior to the gay rights
movement, or live in small towns or rural areas of the United States, or
are members of an ethnic, religious, or racial minority group that stig-
matizes homosexuality more than even the mainstream culture does,
their relationship may be wholly invisible to others. Moreover, in particular moments a male couple may deliberately choose to become invisible to avoid rejection, ridicule, harassment, or physical violence, passing simply as two straight men. That is, just as passing as straight has
helped many a gay boy survive childhood and adolescence, a gay male
couple's passing as two straight men, by momentarily making the status
of their relationship invisible, can be an adaptive survival skill when the
couple finds itself in situations where they may be physically harmed or
psychologically harassed if they are perceived as a same-sex couple. Un-

like other discriminated minority groups who cannot hide their identifying characteristic, gay couples often can choose to keep their sexual orientations and their relationship invisible.[2]

Such invisibility is harmful psychologically because it provides a breeding ground for shame. The invisibility of homosexuality and of same-sex relationships is a dramatic example of how social context not only influences individual behavior but also shapes the self-concept in damaging ways. The mainstream culture, by and large homophobic, prefers not to see evidence of homosexuality. Until he comes out, the gay male takes on an invisible status, taking care not to call attention to that aspect of his identity. Such social oppression corrodes his self-image, as the gay man internalizes the inferior, marginalized status that the culture wishes to impose on him (Hancock, 2000). Shame is the high psychic cost to the gay individual for keeping up appearances and remaining invisible. "Coming out" and refusing to be invisible is the first step toward reducing the shame. Coming out, although it appears to be a discrete event, is a continuous, lifelong process. Not only does the gay individual have to tell many persons continuously as he ages, he may have to "remind" the people he has already told! For example, after coming out to their families, single gay men work out all sorts of arrangements with their families in terms of how openly their homosexuality will be acknowledged. Even after gay sons have come out to the family, there may be an unstated agreement never to speak of it again. Because of lingering homophobia, the gay son is often as uncomfortable as his family in talking more about his homosexuality, so he tacitly accepts the family's policy of "don't ask, don't tell" even though the secret is already out.

Some gay men wait until they become involved in a relationship to come out to their families, using the fact that they are now partnered to help legitimize their homosexuality. In some families, this tactic works.

---

[2] Because secrecy about one's sexual orientation is technically possible, the U.S. military could seriously propose and implement a policy toward homosexuals of "don't ask, don't tell." Most of the American public assumes that, if there are any military men who are gay, they are most certainly single; yet, some do have coupled but closeted relationships. Under current administration guidelines for the military, one's homosexual orientation must be kept secret, and, by implication, any same-sex relationships must be kept covert. If a serviceman reveals his homosexual orientation, his "telling" can be grounds for discharge.

For example, the Jewish mother of another patient, Henry, was so happy that her son was no longer single that she readily accepted both her son's homosexuality and his companion when Henry announced both in one visit home. She told him later that she had felt more sadness because he was alone than over the fact that he was gay. So strong was her emphasis on family life, she lobbied for the couple to adopt children. For other families, however, accepting a homosexual son who is single is easier than acknowledging his relationship with another man. Bringing a man home and introducing him as one's partner can be a blatant violation of the family's "don't ask, don't tell" contract. These families tacitly accept that their son is gay, but they don't want to see tangible evidence of it in the form of the son's romantic partner.

Finally, a gay couple whose relationship has enjoyed general support by the family can still experience invisibility or marginalization. Such marginalization can occur quite suddenly and unexpectedly. For example, 10 years into his relationship, one of the authors was asked by his sister not to bring his partner to a weekend family reunion. The partner had long been ostensibly accepted by the family and had been included for years in family functions. The trigger for the reemergence of the family's homophobia was that the author's sister had a teenaged son who wanted to invite his girlfriend of 6 months to the family gathering. The nephew was worried about what the girlfriend might think if his uncle brought his partner. While one may (or may not) appreciate the nephew's discomfort, for the boy's mother to ask her brother to leave his spouse-equivalent at home was, essentially, a request for her brother's relationship to go underground for the weekend. (Imagine a married son's receiving a similar request from his family to leave his wife at home. The incident, in fact, made the family dynamics tense: the author confronted his sister, and neither he nor his partner attended the family reunion. Although his sister later apologized and was forgiven, the incident has obviously not been forgotten!) On the other hand, the author and his partner were pleasantly surprised one Christmas several years later when the author's mother, who is very skilled in handicrafts, made individual quilts for everyone in her immediate family (her children, their spouses, and her grandchildren). The author's partner got one. What would have been a minor event if the author had been married to a woman became a heart-warming celebration. To this day, that quilt is a symbolic, visible marker that the partner had become a bona fide in-law.

THE START OF A REVOLUTION:
MALE COUPLES BECOME MORE VISIBLE

Although statistically rare compared to heterosexual couples in society, gay male couples are no longer entirely invisible to the general public. Indeed, the phenomenon of gay male couples living openly together over the past three decades is, historically speaking, nothing short of revolutionary. Still, the concept of a male couple remains very much a radical idea, not only for mainstream society but for male couples themselves as they struggle to form and maintain relationships without the advantages of culturally available scripts or models, without the use of traditional boundaries, without the legal and economic benefits of marriage, and without society's full valuing of these relationships.

In the last half of the 20th century, two major sociocultural events occurred that facilitated the extraordinary development of gay couples living openly in the United States. The first, of course, was the gay rights movement. An underground homosexual subculture had begun to coalesce during World War II, when isolated homosexuals found one another and began to develop a "psychological identity as a member of a deviant sexual group" (Bem, 1993). Although homosexuality was considered shameful by the mainstream culture and by homosexuals themselves, these "sexual outlaws" (Rechy, 1977) bonded together to form a tentative group identity as subversives and to reduce their social isolation. But in 1969 with the Stonewall Rebellion, the gay subculture began to be transformed from a secret community to a more public minority group seeking recognition, if not acceptance, by the mainstream culture. Many lesbian and gay activists advocated for a rejection of majority norms. In the gay rights movement, homosexual men and women developed an "oppositional consciousness that an otherized group needs if it is ever to construct a viable identity" (Bem, 1993, p. 172).

The gay rights movement was singularly instrumental in helping gay individuals develop psychologically healthier identities and begin to live more openly as gay individuals in mainstream society. One wonders whether without this political movement the professions of psychiatry and psychology would have ever officially depathologized homosexuality as a mental disorder—as they did in 1973 and 1975, respectively (Bayer, 1987). Afterward, the clinical term "homosexual" began to give way to the more affirmative term "gay" in public discourse, as exemplified in the mid-1980s when *The New York Times* ("all the news that's fit to print") finally allowed the word "gay" in its hallowed news columns. This shift in language also helped gay people feel better about themselves and able to proclaim a gay identity infused with pride, instead of having to hide a supposedly pathological identity cloaked in shame. But, as we have already noted, the gay rights movement initially did nothing at all to recognize or validate gay couples.

The second major sociocultural event that did propel at least some gay couples out of the closet was the AIDS epidemic. Before AIDS, the gay rights movement had helped gay individuals feel entitled to the same pursuits as straight men, including the pursuit of long-term relationships. Gay men had begun quietly forming coupled relationships in increasing numbers in the 1970s and 1980s, as documented by David McWhirter and Andrew Mattison's book *The Male Couple*, published in 1984 just as the AIDS epidemic was beginning. But these relationships were, for the most part, closeted. It took the AIDS crisis to bring male couples to the public's attention.

Just as the Stonewall Rebellion had brought homosexual individuals out of the closet and into the public's mind, AIDS served to publicize male couples. The mass media ran stories on how AIDS was affecting male couples, stories that also brought these couples to the attention of other male couples. Almost overnight, male couples had a few visible role models and also got the first empathy ever from the general public. As Andrew Sullivan (1996) has written, "The victimization of gay men by a disease paradoxically undercut their victimization by a culture. There was no longer a need to kick them when they were already down" (p. 56). Although the AIDS crisis may have caused some single uninfected gay men to retreat in their individual development as gay men, prompting some to go back into the closet or to become celibate (Isay, 1989), for gay men already coupled—whether they were dealing directly with AIDS or not—the AIDS crisis caused their relationships to feel less invisible.

At first, in responding to AIDS, society's mainstream institutions did not acknowledge gay men's partners, as exemplified by hospital staffs not allowing the partner of an AIDS patient to have access to him or to be involved in his care. As the epidemic spread, however, hospitals began to recognize these relationships and to include the partner in the care of the AIDS patient. For example, St. Vincent's Hospital was one of the first medical centers in New York City to recognize the unique psychosocial needs of men who had lost their partners to AIDS. The hospital formed special bereavement groups, which for the first time recognized widowed gay men as spouse-equivalents (Greenan, 1987). Shernoff (1997) has more recently documented the experience of gay widowers.

Moreover, at the start of the AIDS epidemic, the gay community itself did not adequately acknowledge the gay couple as a social entity. As late as 1986, the Gay Men's Health Crisis (GMHC), a progressive social services agency formed by activists in New York City's gay community to cope with AIDS, seemed not to recognize the gay male couple in its otherwise extensive array of mental health services. GMHC split the couple up into different therapies, further rendering gay couples invisible. Persons with AIDS (PWAs) were referred to supportive therapy groups with one another; the partners of PWAs were referred to separate care-partner groups with other care-partners. Years later, multiple couple groups were instituted, which helped the couple face AIDS as a family unit rather than as two separate individuals.

Like GMHC, the gay subculture itself—with its heavy emphasis on individual freedom and autonomy, youth, physical beauty, and permissiveness to act on one's sexual impulses—has not always been "couple friendly." More currently, the trends for some gay couples to hold commitment ceremonies, to push for legal rights to marry, and to adopt children have produced a strong backlash from those sectors of the gay community who view these trends as mimicking heterosexist institutions and values (Warner, 1999). As Harold Kooden (2000) has written, gay men often seem to be saying to nongay society: "We have different rules on how to live and your rules don't fit us" (pp. 130–131). Today it remains common for a young gay man to react with astonishment when he hears that two gay men have been together for as long as 4 years and to be thoroughly incredulous when he hears about relationships that have lasted 15 years or more.

Despite current society's discomfort and now legalized prejudice against same-sex relationships (officially enacted into the U.S. statutory code in 1999 as the Defense of Marriage Act, which defined legal marriage as existing only between opposite-sex individuals), and despite marginalizing experiences ranging from being socially snubbed to being physically beaten, same-sex coupling shows no sign of abating. Some writers have commented that the persistent robustness of homosexuality across all cultures and all historical eras, despite strong societal sanctions and severe punishments, implies that homosexuality must be a biologically natural variant of sexual expression (Davison, 1991). In a similar vein, we marvel at how gay men persist in forming and maintaining long-term same-sex relationships, breaching some of society's strongest rules and prohibitions. Just as all individuals have a strong biological impulse to express themselves sexually, whatever their sexual orientation, individuals have strong needs to attach to others and to form intimate relationships. As John Bowlby (1979) has written, attachment phenomena are natural and alive "from the cradle to the grave." Moreover, as we shall see, attachment phenomena operate in same-sex romantic relationships just as they do in long-term heterosexual ones (Mohr, 1999).

In his theory of personality development over the lifespan, Erik Erikson (1950) has written that once a person achieves a stable individual identity in adolescence and young adulthood, the next developmental task is to form a close romantic relationship. Erikson had heterosexuals in mind as he wrote his theory, but the basic stages apply equally to gay men. Green, Bettinger, and Zacks (1996), after reviewing a number of studies that demonstrate the desire of gay men to be in a dating or committed relationship, conclude that "the idea that most gay men prefer being unattached is simply a myth" (p. 214). In addition, following Eriksonian theory that after becoming coupled there is a desire for generativity, which for most heterosexuals is most commonly expressed by having children, we have seen in recent years a rise in the number of male couples pursuing the adoption of children or arranging surrogate births, a societal phenomenon unheard of just a few years ago.

Same-sex unions and families share, as well as defy, traditional notions of couples and families. Similarities and differences between heterosexual and male same-sex couples need to be recognized, and couple therapy needs to accommodate the differences. This book is a beginning guide for family therapists on how to do that.

ISSUES THAT MAKE GAY MALE COUPLES DIFFERENT

Along with demonstrating the problems of invisibility and the lack of social support male couples typically receive, the case of Kurt and Rob exemplifies two other issues gay male couples can present to family therapists. Many male couples choose to be sexually nonmonogamous (Blumstein & Schwartz, 1983), a choice that defies traditional notions of being coupled and may unsettle traditionally trained family therapists. For nonmonogamous male couples, the commitment to the primary relationship is usually about emotional fidelity, attachment, and dependability, not sexual faithfulness. In fact, these three aspects of gay male couples—their invisibility, their lack of social support, their frequent nonmonogamy—set them apart from heterosexual marriages and produce conditions that increase the difficulty for the male couple to put a boundary around itself. Couples and families require boundaries around them so that both they and others can differentiate themselves as separate social structures with their own rules and organization (Minuchin, 1974).

A fourth difference of gay male couples, also exemplified by Kurt and Rob, is their unique difficulties in emotional and relational functioning, as compared to heterosexual couples. The case of Kurt and Rob illustrated problems in self-disclosing their feelings, expressing intimacy and affection, and working through conflicts and differences without dominance-based tactics. Mainstream culture privileges and reinforces "alpha" male behavior, regardless of sexual orientation. Most men are acculturated to be strong rather than weak, independent rather than dependent, aggressive rather than passive, noncompromising rather than accommodating, and rational and problem-solving rather than emotional. The language of business and government contains warlike, winner-take-all terminology that reveals the thinking that supports male behavior ("hostile takeovers," "bull and bear markets"). American culture does not reward accommodating behavior between men, and capitalism encourages aggressive behavior toward others in the pursuit of profits. For men in the affairs of the world to exhibit softer "feminine" behaviors—such as accommodation, compromise, or empathy, especially in dealing with other men—violates society's standards for the male gender role.

Just as many husbands in a capitalistic society have trouble turning off male gender-role standards when they try relating intimately to their wives, many gay men have the same issue, only magnified, because their attempt to create intimacy is with another man. That is, a man's homosexuality does not make him immune to the strong forces of male gender acculturation. Indeed, it is precisely because gay males growing up become so sensitized about appearing needy, feminine, or "sissy" that they may find it difficult to be vulnerable with their male adult partners. Having experienced vulnerability in their early relationships with families and peers, and responding to that vulnerability by developing emotional self-reliance over many years, they may find that intimacy with another man becomes a real challenge, with the possibility that one might be humiliated all over again.

Our clinical experience suggests that, whatever difficulties married men may have in being emotionally sensitive (even vulnerable) to their wives, the difficulties a man has in being emotionally vulnerable to another man are much more formidable. An intimate relationship with a woman is one of the few culturally sanctioned places where a man may be emotionally vulnerable. That is, society renders it acceptable, if not desirable, for a man to be vulnerable and emotionally expressive in an intimate opposite-sex relationship. Even though some men may still find it difficult to be vulnerable with a woman, we submit that it is far more difficult for the average man to be emotionally vulnerable to another man, not only because of society's homophobic judgments about same-sex intimacy but also because of the gay man's resistance to placing himself emotionally in the hands of another man.

Some authors (Green et al., 1996) have suggested that gay men are "gendered differently" from straight men and may have, by implication, less difficulty with emotional and relational functioning. Research has shown that gay men are, on average as compared to straight men, more androgynous (Kurdek, 1987). Androgynous individuals show a combination of both male-associated self-assertion and female-associated relatedness. Gay men who are more androgynous may in fact be better equipped to sustain emotional connections. In research on nonclinical populations by Green at al. (1996) that compared lesbian, gay male, and heterosexual couples, male couples reported higher levels of cohesion and flexibility in their relationships than did heterosexual couples (lesbian couples reported the highest levels of all). Contrary to gender role theory, male couples were not the most disengaged of the three groups, but rather heterosexual couples were. Whether their possibly greater androgyny or lesser reliance on rigid gender roles accounts for their higher level of relational functioning is a question that awaits future research.

However, the men we see in treatment, whether straight or gay, often seem to have considerable difficulty in relational functioning, possibly due to their strong gender training. Such difficulties with intimacy become multiplied when the relationship is composed of two men. In brief, the most common struggles we see in male couples are how to accommodate to the other's needs (without suffering a loss of face) and how to sustain over time a loving relationship that combines emotional intimacy with sexual passion. These struggles are, of course, also commonly seen in heterosexual couples. However, differences exist in how these struggles get resolved. With heterosexual couples, social constraints exist for them to work out their differences and remain together, whereas among male couples, at the first sign of conflict, the tendency is to separate. Also, among gay men there is more social acceptability from their subculture for them to find sexual passion outside of the primary relationship.

OUR MODEL: MODIFYING STRUCTURAL FAMILY THERAPY FOR MALE COUPLES

The case example of Rob and Kurt introduces some ways in which our work, based on Salvador Minuchin's (1974; Minuchin & Fishman, 1981) three-stage model of structural family therapy (joining, enactments, unbalancing), is noticeably different when applied to gay male couples. First, therapists must demonstrate unusually strong joining during the initial stage of therapy—beginning in the very first session— by respectfully regarding the male couple as a social unit having as much legitimacy as a heterosexual couple. Given that many male couples have internalized their marginalized status and may expect therapists to judge, pathologize, or discredit their relationship, therapists must go out of their way to demonstrate acceptance during the early stages of therapy. This strong joining, in and of itself, begins to form a boundary around the couple that validates them as a legitimate social structure.

Examples of strong joining with a male couple include (1) referring to the men as "a couple" from the outset, just as a heterosexual man and woman would be regarded; (2) recognizing established differences between male couples and heterosexual couples by asking male couples in a matter-of-fact manner whether they are monogamous, the decision making that underlay that, and what the current rules are; (3) asking how and in what ways the relationship is respected by their families and friends; (4) asking specifically what anniversary date the partners celebrate and why, since few gay couples have had any sort of ceremony that marks the "official" start of their relationship, yet almost all gay couples have some sort of anniversary marker they do celebrate; (5) directly expressing empathy when they describe incidents where the relationship is rendered invisible by others; (6) taking a nonpathologizing stance when they discuss such an issue as nonmonogamy, which would almost certainly be labeled as a serious problem by family therapists working with married heterosexual couples (Lusterman, 1995; Pittman, 1987); (7) inquiring whether the couple has had, or intends to have, a commitment ceremony; and (8) if the couple does not have children, asking if they plan to. Asking these questions indicates to the male couple that the therapist takes them seriously.

Second, in working with male couples who lack a strong intimate connection with each other and have difficulty with emotional expressiveness, during the middle and later stages of treatment (enactments and unbalancing), the therapist must work actively toward helping each member of the couple become more personally vulnerable and revealing, and to become more responsive to the other's vulnerabilities. Most gay men have been shamed about their core identities, their vulnerabilities, and their needs for same-sex support, affection, and love. Couple therapy can be a corrective emotional experience in which each man's needs can be directly expressed to his male partner, with the partner expected to be highly attentive and responsive.

In this regard, our therapeutic approach challenges gender stereotypes about how men are supposed to behave with one another. A loving, coupled relationship can provide a relational experience in which secrecy about one's core being is no longer so necessary. A gay man often grows up believing he has only himself to rely on. This belief, while perhaps adaptive in surviving childhood and adolescence, interferes with developing healthy partnered relationships, and in couple therapy this belief needs to be actively challenged.

In sum, in strongly joining with the couple, we show respect and empathy for the marginalizing and stigmatizing experiences many male couples have endured, yet in later stages of treatment we challenge them to make their relationships more fulfilling generally and more intimate particularly. One function of couple therapy with gay men is to help them tolerate a higher level of emotional expressiveness with each other without resorting to stereotypically male-based strategies of dominance, intimidation, shaming, and stonewalling. In challenging the male couple to experiment with new, more affiliative interpersonal behaviors, the therapist creates a treatment environ that introduces novelty. We normalize—treat as normal—the men's needs for a sense of dependency, closeness, and nurturance. Treatment in this respect is a political act, challenging societal norms that the heterosexual family is the preferred (if not the only) family constellation. The therapist creates an opportunity for gay men to experiment with nontraditional, less stereotypical behaviors associated with being male in U.S. culture.[3]

THERAPISTS' ATTITUDES

As family therapists who work with gay male couples, we must examine continuously our own attitudes toward homosexuality, especially our homophobia and heterosexist bias, which we ourselves cannot help but acquire growing up in U.S. culture. Even therapists who are themselves gay and who claim to be entirely supportive of same-sex relationships can unknowingly project an antigay bias if they are uncomfortable witnessing, and encouraging, same-sex intimacy. No one—including psychotherapists—grows up in our culture without internalizing some of the culture's homophobia, heterosexism, and discomfort with behavior that is "gender-inappropriate" (behavior that does not conform to gender-role expectations). We have met psychotherapists who claim to work effectively with gay clients in individual psychotherapy yet persist in seeking out answers to the origins of the client's homosexuality, imposing on the patient the question of how it is he became gay even though the question is of little interest to him, a line of inquiry that implicitly pathologizes him. Although these therapists are in principle gay-affirmative, their techniques are subtly homophobic. On several occasions we have experienced blatant antigay bias when presenting our work with gay couples at professional meetings. Once, following a videotaped presentation of the case described in Chapter 7, in which an emotionally moving dialogue occurs between a male couple, one of whom is dying of AIDS, a psychiatrist in the audience asked with the utmost seriousness, "In your work with this couple, what did you do about the men's homosexuality?"

The point here is that, however well-intentioned and effective gay-

---

[3] Obviously, our model also has implications for couple therapy with heterosexual couples, where straight men often need to be pushed to experiment with behaviors new to them.

affirmative psychotherapists may be in treating gay individual clients, conducting couple treatment with two men in a same-sex relationship forces therapists to confront their own biases in ways that individual therapy does not do. We have discussed how some families of gay sons can conveniently ignore their child's homosexuality as long as he is not involved in a serious relationship. But once the son falls in love and begins an open partnership with another man, the family's covert homophobia can emerge full force. Witnessing their gay son show affection to another man, seeing the two men together in the same bed, or having the son's partner attend family events can test the limits of their acceptance. For couple therapists who believe sincerely that they are not homophobic, who claim no special allegiance to a heterosexist value system, and who believe that gender roles do constrain all people, discomfort can still occur as they watch—let alone, encourage—two men in their offices to be tender, dependent, or affectionate with each other. And yet this is what we have come to believe that couple work with gay men is often about.

In our experience developing a therapeutic model with male couples, men—particularly those who have been strongly acculturated to the traditional male role—need to be prompted, either through encouragement, permission, or direct challenge by the therapist, to behave with greater tenderness, compassion, and affection toward one another. These interventions by the therapist "unbalance" the couple and create novelty for the men. Some couple therapists will undoubtedly feel anxious intervening in this way with two men, even though these same therapists may routinely promote greater intimacy in their work with opposite-sex couples.

CHAPTER TWO

Implications for
Man-to-Man Closeness
from Growing Up Gay

In our clinical experience one theme that links a variety of problems couples present in therapy is a fundamental conflict about how close (or distant) they desire to be with each other. To what degree does each partner want mutuality, interpersonal contact, and emotional connection, as opposed to autonomy, independence, and separation? Mature intimacy requires both a capacity to be independent and separate and a capacity to be close to the other emotionally and to acknowledge needs for attachment, connectedness, and dependency.

All couples negotiate closeness and distance in their relationships, and gay male couples are no different. But, for reasons explored in this chapter, male couples in therapy frequently have unique difficulties in closeness/distance regulation, in allowing dependent bonds to form, and in maintaining emotional connections over time. Although gay males desire emotionally intimate relationships with other men (Green et al., 1996), they are often ambivalent about closeness, partly because of male gender socialization (which conditions males to become proficient in emotional self-sufficiency and independence) and partly because of distinctively negative developmental experiences many gay men have had with other males. These early childhood experiences may make close connection with other men unfamiliar, awkward, or difficult. Many gay men—more so than with straight men—learn over time that it is simply too risky to reveal one's emotional vulnerability to another man.

We believe these early socialization experiences lead gay males to overdevelop their separateness, a defensive overvaluing of personal autonomy that subsequently creates problems in adult interpersonal relationships, where greater closeness is required. In the first half of this chapter, we review theories that speak to the dual needs of every individual to relate intimately with another person *and* to maintain one's separateness. Both needs endure over one's entire lifetime, from "cradle to grave," as Bowlby has said. We review Bowen's concept of differentiation and Bowlby's concept of attachment and suggest they are parallel accounts of the same phenomenon, the continuous interplay between the needs for autonomy and connection. Both Bowen and Bowlby have postulated that during childhood and adolescence individuals acquire relatively fixed expectations for closeness and distance in adult intimate relationships. Finally, we examine the role of gender acculturation in setting up "appropriate" levels of distance and closeness for men in personal relationships. In the second half of the chapter, we look more specifically at the early development of gay men through these lenses, with a particular eye toward understanding how they regulate closeness and distance in adult romantic relationships.

DIFFERENTIATION OF SELF

Despite an inordinate valuing of individual autonomy by American culture and in psychological theory, the basic human tendency is to seek *both* autonomy and connection throughout one's entire life (Rank, 1929; Angyl, 1951; Bakan, 1966). That is, all human beings desire autonomy from, as well as attachment to and communion with, other living beings outside the self. In relating to the external object, the individual has a transcendent emotional or spiritual experience he cannot have on his own. The dual needs to be separate and to be connected are deep-seated, persist throughout an individual's lifetime, and are not necessarily at odds. In fact, having both needs satisfied, according to these personality theorists, constitutes the essence of being fully human.

The dual needs to be separate and to be connected are reflected in family systems theorists' understanding of intimate relationships. Murray

Bowen (1966) combined both concepts—the need for separateness and the need for emotional connection—in his seminal concept of differentiation. He argued that the individual's primary task from birth on was the "differentiation of self," which is not solely about achieving independence and autonomy (as the word "differentiation" implies) but something more comprehensive and far more difficult for most people: *Differentiation is ultimately about being "an authentic self-in-relation."* Because the need for emotional connection is so strong, however, many individuals never fully develop their autonomous, authentic selves.

Bowen valued the individual's ability to be autonomous (to think rationally rather than to react emotionally) over the capacity to be relational, since without moderate levels of individual autonomy mature intimacy with others is simply not possible. In adult relationships formed by poorly differentiated individuals, intimacy and closeness are limited, because the individuals show either too much or too little emotional reaction to one another. Emotional reactivity and emotional cutoffs were, according to Bowen, cardinal signs that the individual needed to differentiate more, either in learning to be more separate or learning to remain connected. As Schnarch (1997) has suggested, in poorly differentiated couples each person's level of self-disclosure is overly dependent on the responsiveness of the partner.

In his emphasis on the primacy of the individual's autonomous functioning, Bowen perhaps gave insufficient attention to the relational context that enables individual authenticity to develop in the first place and later to be maintained and allowed to grow. Differentiation is not just about achieving individual autonomy at all costs but also is about maintaining a deep emotional connection to the other without losing one's self (Schnarch, 1997). Healthy dyadic relationships are those where both parties respect and value the other's core self and its boundaries while simultaneously sustaining an emotional connection. Remaining true to one's real self in relational functioning is one ideal, but so is maintaining strong connections while being true to one's self. Losing one's connections for the sake of autonomy can be just as awful experientially and developmentally as losing one's autonomy for the sake of maintaining one's connections.

Although differentiation of self within relationships is theoretically a lifelong process that begins in infancy and continues until death, most people acquire a basic level of differentiation by young adulthood as they separate from their families of origin and form their own separate identity. This basic level of differentiation then functions as a semi-permanent, relatively stable trait that guides one's subsequent experiences in close relationships outside the family. Bowen (1978) believed that, in forming coupled relationships, individuals were attracted to others with a level of differentiation similar to their own. Moreover, it proves difficult for most people to raise their basic level of differentiation by any significant degree once adulthood is reached (Schnarch, 1997), even when different stages of the life cycle (Erikson, 1950; Carter & McGoldrick, 1998) require it. Psychiatric symptoms often emerge at transition points where the relative degrees of connection or autonomy need to shift. For example, in a healthy resolution of one's identity crisis during adolescence and young adulthood as the individual separates from the family of origin, the need for autonomy is more front and center as the need for familial connection recedes. In forming romantic attachments, connection with a new other comes to the fore, while the other need—maintaining one's autonomous self—recedes to the background. Both needs are ubiquitous. Though at any given moment or stage of life one need may be more prominent, the other will need to be satisfied eventually.

In formulating structural family therapy, Salvador Minuchin (1974) has elucidated ideas about relational functioning that in many ways parallel Bowen's. Differentiation of self in Bowen's theory is akin to boundaries in Minuchin's theory. Boundary making and boundary regulation are key concepts in how Minuchin conceptualizes family systems, describing the extremes as either "enmeshed" or "disengaged." An enmeshed system is a family or couple with poorly delineated boundaries between the individuals, where there is too much emotional engagement and too little autonomy. Individuals are continuously and intrusively into each other's affairs, with the family members unable to respect boundaries and to tolerate separateness, either one's own or the other's.[1] A disengaged system is one in which boundaries are too rigid, where there is too much individual autonomy and too little connection. A disengaged system is characterized by emotionally distant individuals who appear disinterested in the other's affairs, value boundaries at the expense of emotional connection, and

---

[1] Enmeshment may entail three separate components—closeness/caregiving, openness of communication, and intrusiveness—with only intrusiveness being pathological (Green et al., 1996; Werner, Green, Greenberg, Browne, & McKenna, 2001).

minimally engage each other. A healthy system, according to Minuchin, is neither enmeshed nor disengaged but rather has clear boundaries that are also permeable. For Bowen, a couple's regulation of closeness and distance is largely a function of the two individuals' levels of differentiation. For Minuchin, it is a function of the individuals' abilities to create and maintain boundaries as well as, for flexibility's sake, to permeate them periodically.

In coupled relationships, each individual strives to maintain some preferred balance of autonomy and connection. That is, everyone, when feeling too isolated or disconnected, will initiate social contact of some sort. Similarly all individuals, when feeling too close or hemmed in, will initiate a withdrawal of contact. But the thresholds for seeking closeness and distance vary from individual to individual. Problems emerge in couples when the two individuals are persistently out of sync, sometimes becoming played out in the classic dance of the pursuer/distancer, first described by Fogarty (1979). Nichols and Minuchin (1999) have noted the circular, complementary cycles of closeness–distance regulation in which couples engage and which can escalate into extreme polarization. When one individual pursues more closeness than the other is comfortable with, the other distances, an action that prompts the first individual to pursue closeness even more, which causes the other to distance even more, and so on. Minuchin has argued that the goal for couples is flexibility and permeability—to be sometimes close and connected, at other times distant and separate, and to tolerate those times when one's partner isn't so accommodating.

ATTACHMENT THEORY

It seems clear that individuals differ in how much closeness and distance they prefer in intimate one-on-one relationships. How do these preferences develop in the first place? John Bowlby's (1969/1982, 1973) attachment theory offers one account for individual differences in closeness seeking and distance seeking that develop in infancy and appear to persist into adolescence and adulthood. The original attachment bond is formed between the infant and the primary caregiver, usually the mother or mother figure. Attachment bonds, as distinct from other types of social relationships, have four unique characteristics: "proximity maintenance," "separation protest," "secure base," and "safe haven."

As we will see, the same four functions of attachment operate in intimate romantic adult relationships.

When mother–infant attachment goes well, the primary caregiver serves as a secure base from which the infant explores the environment. The infant continuously monitors the mother's proximity and availability. When threatened, the infant turns to her for comfort and resists becoming completely separated from her. Good mothering grants the infant independence as the child requires it, neither allowing the infant more independence than can be handled nor forcing independence when the child isn't ready. The good mother is attuned to what the child seems to need. Autonomy and attachment, according to Bowlby, go hand in hand. It is precisely the infant's feeling of security with the attachment figure that allows it to develop a zestful sense of autonomy and exploration. Without secure attachment, real autonomy and authentic individuality cannot fully develop.[2]

Similar to psychoanalytic theory[3] Bowlby held that infants, based on experiences with their early attachment figures, develop rudimentary "internal working models" to predict the behavior of attachment figures in later life. Securely attached infants develop a working model or internal representation that subsequent attachment figures will be available and responsive when needed. Securely attached individuals are not threatened by physical and emotional closeness because their working model of relationships includes the expectation that the other will respect one's own boundaries, one's core self, and one's need for autonomy. There is consequently no need to fear the other's proximity. In other words, the securely attached individual is comfortable with both

---

[2] In toddlers, striking behavioral differences in attachment styles emerged when they were separated from the mother and left in a "strange situation" without her (Ainsworth, Blehar, Waters, & Wall, 1978). From studying attachment behavior in the laboratory and in the home, Ainsworth and Bowlby specified three types of attachment bonds. A *securely attached* infant registers protest when separated from the mother, is soothed fairly easily when she returns, and within a few moments resumes play. *Insecurely attached* infants show one of two different patterns of behavior. The *avoider* subtype does not protest the separation and barely notices the mother when she returns, appears indifferent to her, and stays focused on solitary play. Other insecurely attached infants—those subtyped *ambivalent/anxious*—fret during and after the mother's leave-taking, alternate between accepting and rejecting her attempts to provide comfort, and find it difficult to resume autonomous play.

[3] See Fonagy (1999) for a comparison of psychoanalytic and attachment theories.

autonomy and connection and moves fairly easily into either state. In contrast, insecurely attached adults react quickly when they perceive the attachment figure as either too close (insecure/avoidant subtype) or too distant (insecure/ambivalent subtype). When avoiders sense encroachment by the attachment figure, they seek distance. Ambivalent/ anxious types are particularly sensitive to abandonment; when they sense distance, they may initially attempt to distance themselves but ultimately respond by pursuing or clinging.

Over the past two decades, social, developmental, and clinical psychologists have applied attachment theory to romantic love (Allen & Land, 1999; Hazen & Zeifman, 1999; Collins & Read, 1990; Feeney, 1999; Johnson, 1999), beginning with Hazan and Shaver (1987), who found support for the existence of the same three attachment styles in adult relationships.[4] This research is exciting as well as controversial: Is attachment style stable over the lifespan? How does new experience with significant others change attachment organization? To what degree is attachment more a function of individuals or of specific relationships? Is it ever possible for a new relationship to create its own fresh attachment dynamics with little regard to past experience?

Some research supports Bowlby's hypothesis that individuals behave in accordance with their internal working models, or beliefs about how relationships are supposed to work. Acting on those beliefs, individuals play a crucial role in inducing the responsiveness and support they actually receive from significant others. That is, secure individuals expect enjoyable and supportive encounters with others, and they behave in a manner that elicits such experiences. Insecure persons expect less satisfying encounters and may behave in ways that interfere with having more supportive experiences with their romantic partners (Thompson, 1999). This phenomenon, we believe, is particularly at work in gay men's romantic relationships. Because many gay men do not expect another man to be responsive and supportive to him emotionally, they often behave in distancing ways that make their expectation come true.

---

[4] Of course, in applying attachment theory to adult romantic relationships, the reciprocal nature of the relationship means dual roles for the partners and makes the adult–adult scenario more complex than the parent–child scenario: "Each mate uses the other as an attachment figure and source of security; each also serves as an attachment figure and provider of security to the other" (Hazan & Zeifman, 1999).

MALE ACCULTURATION AND MALE COUPLES

As a final complication in closeness/distance regulation, the culture values autonomy and connection differently as a function of gender. According to gender role theory (Basow, 1992), men are supposed to be relatively more independent, emotionally self-reliant, and more autonomous overall, while women are supposed to be more oriented to the needs of others, more emotionally sensitive, and more connected and relational overall. While Bowen seemed to give greater value in both genders to autonomy over dependency (and thinking over feeling), Bowlby on the other hand viewed attachment and emotional dependency as healthy and desirable, regardless of gender. That is, attachment and dependency are not infantile states that either males or females should necessarily outgrow. Minuchin (1974; Minuchin, Lee, & Simon, 1996) has also been more balanced in terms of which state is more desirable: Healthy relationships require both individual separation and interpersonal connectedness.[5] In less healthy relationships partners can become polarized, often along gender lines. Thus, in heterosexual relationships it is often the man who becomes the voice of separation and the woman who becomes the voice of connection. In healthier couples, regardless of sexual orientation, there is less polarization and more flexibility in roles: The partner who wanted distance yesterday is ready for closeness today. Problems occur when the partners get stuck in the same, complementary roles all the time.

What happens to closeness–distance regulation in gay male couples? Because they are both men, should we expect to find two chronic distancers, as Krestan and Bepko (1980) suggested, based on gender role theory? As Mohr (1999) and Green et al. (1996) have documented, it's not that simple. Closeness–distance dynamics operate in same-sex

---

[5] In each of these theoretical perspectives, it should be emphasized again that autonomy and connection are reciprocally dependent on each other. Autonomy has no meaning without a social referent; an individual becomes autonomous and differentiated *from* someone else and yet remains in relationship with that person. An emotional cutoff (Bowen, 1978), where one or both parties angrily proclaim independence and say they want nothing more from the other, does not produce mature autonomy but rather a counterdependence. An emotional cutoff is just another version of emotional reactivity. Similarly, mature emotional connection or attachment has no meaning without the recognition of two individual, separate selves; otherwise, the connection is pure symbiotic merger and only "one undifferentiated ego mass" (Bowen, 1978).

couples but not always along gender lines. Although we have worked with male couples where both men persistently distance, it is more usual to find one partner seeking closeness and the other seeking distance. In complementary fashion, one man takes up the voice of connectedness while the other takes up the voice of separation. What is distinctive in male couples is that the man who adopts the voice of connectedness may feel shame about his desire for emotional closeness *with a man*. When a straight man wants to connect emotionally with a woman, he may feel shame about his emotional dependency, but he is not violating strong cultural norms about male–female closeness by his desire to feel close to a woman. The gay man, on the other hand, is in a double bind. He wants closeness, but the object is another man. As Johnson and Keren (1996) have written: "Intimacy with another man can provoke a man to feel unmasculine and worthless, whereas distance may render him lonely and depressed. For such men, sexual orientation is experienced as a perpetual double bind, permitting no comfortable solution and causing havoc in their couple relationships" (p. 244).

In the next section as we apply attachment theory to gay men's relationships, our interest is in two separate areas. First, what happens in attachment dynamics between the boy and his parents, especially the father, when the boy is discovering his homosexuality in childhood and adolescence? Even if he has developed previously a healthy internal working model of relationships—that he himself is lovable no matter what and that his attachment figure can be counted on if needed—can he actually turn to his parental attachment figures for support during the process when he is discovering his homosexuality? We speculate that most parents are not able to be empathically responsive to the gay youth when he is struggling with a culturally deviant sexual identity. This leaves him, at least for a while, with an insecure tie to his primary attachment figures. He may develop a predisposition to distance from significant others and/or an ambivalent attitude toward close relationships, even if he had previously enjoyed responsive parenting.

Second, we are interested in the types of attachment bonds adult gay male couples create and maintain with each other. Given that many gay males grow up keeping their emotional lives private from others, are gay male partners able to turn to each other when each needs "a safe haven"? Will the other be responsive? Moreover, when a man is responsive to his partner's emotional needs, can the partner accept the support and empathy? Several theorists have suggested that gay men, particularly those with high degrees of internalized homophobia (Mohr, 1999; Tunnell, 1991), find it difficult "tolerating nourishing relations" with other men (Isay, 1989, p. 60). Mohr (1999) has examined attachment bonds in same-sex couples and suggests that attachment bonds operate similarly to those in heterosexual couples—with an important exception. He notes that the insecure/avoidant attachment style (the "distancer" in adult relationships) is empirically associated with internalized homophobia, which he suggests interferes with tolerating closeness and trust in another man. Mohr's finding makes sense: The greater the shame internalized in being gay, the more likely a man is to distance himself emotionally in close relationships with other men.

THE TRAUMA OF DISCOVERING ONE'S HOMOSEXUALITY

For the most part, gay men have not been viewed in light of these theories. Yet, we believe these models illuminate how many gay men go about constructing their relational worlds.[6] In these theories, all persons—regardless of gender or sexual orientation—are assumed to have the dual needs of separation and connection. However, gender acculturation and sexual orientation complicate the attainment of these basic needs for gay men.

Gender role theory holds that males are traditionally assumed to have more difficulty with connection and maintaining emotional relationships, given that they are acculturated to be more autonomous, dis-

---

[6] No one knows with any certainty what percentage of the population is homosexual, or, even more perplexing for some, the origins of homosexuality. Based on available research evidence and theory, we take more of an "essentialist" position (Broido, 2000), that sexual orientation is more constitutionally than environmentally determined. Sexual orientation is discovered by the individual as it emerges through fantasies, interests, or actual experiences, which the individual then attributes with meaning. What we especially want to avoid in our discussion applying attachment theory to gay men is that homosexuality represents some sort of "attachment error," that is, that homosexuality is the consequence of a poor attachment between the infant and either the mother or the father. Homosexuality happens pretty much on its own, yet has major ramifications on relationships as everyone reacts to it. We are most interested here in what happens to attachment dynamics in the parent–child bond as the boy is discovering he is attracted to individuals of the same sex.

tant, and separate, first by parents (Chodorow, 1978) and subsequently by societal institutions through gender-role prescriptions (Basow, 1992). The cultural gender-role prescription for males is based on being a strong, separate, and independent individual at all costs. Brannon (1976) has summarized the male role as having four parts: (1) show "no sissy stuff" (the need to be different from females), (2) be the "big wheel" (the need to be superior to others), (3) be the "sturdy oak" (the need to be self-reliant and independent), and (4) give 'em hell (the need to be more powerful than others). The social consequences for young boys who violate this adult Marlboro Man script by showing weakness, dependency, or vulnerability can be swift and severe. As early as age 5, boys are called "girlish," "sissy," or even "fag" and "queer" by their peers and adults. While racial or ethnic slurs about other minority groups are often punished by responsible adults, slurs regarding gender role violations continue to be tolerated. By taunting and shaming the young boy, the culture shapes the boy to conform to its expectations for males.

As Lawrence Kohlberg (1966) and Sandra Bem (1981) have pointed out, however, the boy is not a passive participant in his cultural conditioning. Because he understands cognitively that he is male and as part of his identity development strives to be male-like, he actively participates in his own gender acculturation. If he senses that he is not sufficiently like other males, he may proactively identify male role models and imitate their behavior. His motivation is not simply to become like other males but to differentiate himself from females. Particularly for males, Western culture extracts severe penalties for exhibiting cross-gender behavior. Underlying these limits about what is permissible behavior for males is the culture's strong prejudice against homosexuality and the confounding in the public's mind of male homosexuality versus feminine character traits and behaviors (see box on page 30).

For a homosexual boy who exhibits female-like behaviors and interests—a phenomenon increasingly seen by child psychiatrists and developmental psychologists as a rather normal precursor of an eventual homosexual orientation (American Psychiatric Association, 1994; Bailey & Zucker, 1995, Green, 1987), others significant to the boy usually react with concern and alarm. Peers and parents of the feminized boy make him feel different and alien from other boys, setting up a context for social–emotional isolation. The isolation and alienation, whether imposed by others or himself, may occur long before the boy ever labels

Components of Sexual Identity

In the mind of the public, as in the minds of many psychotherapists, the components of sexual identity have long been confounded as one dimension. Although developmental psychologists and others have recognized at least five separate components of sexual identity—biological sex, gender identity, gender-role characteristics, sexual orientation, and sexual identity (Baslow, 1992; Pillard, 1991)—in everyday life people continue to confuse them. While people can appreciate in the abstract that each is a different construct, they nonetheless assume certain correlations as they observe people in everyday life. In such a simple world, biological males are expected to claim a male gender identity, acquire gender-role characteristics culturally "appropriate" for males, be sexually attracted to the opposite gender, and form a heterosexual identity. Gender-atypical behavior confuses and often upsets many people, from young children to mature adults, as does homosexuality. Moreover, once a deviation occurs in one component of sexual identity, lay people generally expect to find other deviations. That is, once a person is perceived as homosexual, he might also be assumed to be effeminate, or to not be comfortable as a male, or to really prefer to be female (Isay, 1989).

In psychiatry Freud is partly responsible for establishing these simplistic assumptions about sexual identity. Freud gave a psychoanalytic account of how these very different dimensions unfolded all together around the age of 5 and how, by the time of adolescence, were solidified. The young boy, in discovering the biological differences between the sexes, sees his penis as a symbol of his maleness. His love for his mother at around that age becomes eroticized. Different psychoanalytic accounts have been constructed for why the boy takes on male gender characteristics similar to those of the father at this point. In one view, the boy identifies with the father's masculine characteristics in an effort to capture the mother's attention. In another account, the boy views his father as an aggressive competitor for the mother's love. To reduce his anxiety that the father, with his larger physical size and larger penis, can destroy him or his penis, he identifies with the father in a defensive maneuver called identification with the aggressor, taking on the aggressor's presumed masculine gender characteristics. Regardless of the specific dynamics, in Freud's account gender-role characteristics are acquired through an identification with the father. The important point here is that in Freudian theory all dimensions of sexual identity develop in one process simultaneously, albeit in a complex fashion. That is, if the boy "successfully" completes Freud's Oedipal stage, he takes on a male identity, develops male sex-role characteristics, and identifies as heterosexual.

Freud did not believe that childhood upbringing caused either heterosexuality or homosexuality but rather that sexual orientation was determined constitutionally. He does not really explain, in other words, why the young boy is erotically attracted to the mother but instead assumes that opposite-sex attraction is biologically rooted. Richard Isay (1989), in proposing a psychoanalytic account for what happens to homosexual boys during the Oedipal phase of development, also views homosexuality as almost entirely constitutional. In accounting for why many gay individuals also have feminine characteristics, Isay has asserted that the gay boy, in his effort to attract the attention of his father, unconsciously takes on the feminine characteristics of the mother.

himself as homosexual. If the boy shows obvious gender-atypical behavior or other signs that he may possibly be homosexual, parents may try to stamp it out, either by ignoring his behavior or becoming obsessively critical of it. *Either way, parents end up emotionally abandoning or condemning him, at exactly the moment the child needs empathy, support, and reassurance.*

If the boy's cross-gender behavior is so extreme and unremitting that the parents cannot ignore it, and especially if the boy overtly voices his own sexual or gender confusion by actually saying, "I wish I were a girl," the parents may further stigmatize him by sending him to a therapist, who may erroneously diagnose him with gender identity disorder. His behavior may actually be an early natural unfolding of an underlying homosexual orientation (Green, 1987), although that possibility is rarely consoling to parents.

For the boy who may not even understand at this point he is homosexual, such family turmoil is confusing and alienating. As he, and possibly his parents, try to sort out the components of his sexual identity, a rupture is very likely to occur between him and his primary attachment figures, particularly the father.[7] Richard Isay (1989) has provided a vivid and sad account of how the father begins to distance himself from a son who shows gender-atypical behavior and/or erotic interest in the father. The boy himself also initiates distancing behavior from the father out of his own shame. The gay boy's male peers are rarely of help to him during this time. Even if male friends want to be supportive, they generally aren't, else they incur through association the same stigmatization—being labeled queer or sissy themselves. This is often the time when female friends become important to the gay boy (Savin-Williams, 1998), as girls incur less social risk for being his friend.

The point here is that, in a homophobic culture, the homosexual boy is left alone holding an enormous shameful secret he feels cannot be shared. Left to deal with the matter on his own, he is forced to become even more separate and independent than heterosexual boys, who simply do not struggle so intensely with sexual identity issues. This

---

[7] Not all gay boys display feminine behavior or early overt signs that they may be homosexual. Ruptures in attachment dynamics with the father may, in fact, be less serious for them. Yet, masculinized boys who become aware of their erotic attraction to other males quickly adapt to social pressures to keep their real feelings a secret, which can interfere with making deep emotional connections with other men.

sense of separation is not healthy autonomy (in the Bowenian or Bowlby sense) but, more accurately, an isolated loneliness driven by anticipatory shame. Long before he admits to himself that he is homosexual and has begun the process of telling others, which usually does not occur before adolescence or early adulthood, there has already been a rupture between the child and his attachment figures. More specifically, in terms of our interest in gay male couples, the gay boy may develop an internal working model of relationships that he cannot rely on other males—his father or male friends—for protection, nurturance, and solace. Other males are perceived as simply not safe and do not offer a secure base.

In short, the gay male in his early childhood development—before he has developed a gay identity—can undergo traumatic experiences in which his connection with other males is threatened or becomes ruptured. His primary attachments become less secure to him. Even if the homosexual male as an infant had previously developed a healthy internal working model about relationships—a model that he is lovable and that the other will be available and responsive to him—his emerging homosexuality, interpreted in a cultural context that views homosexuality as negative and deviant, may cause him to revise his working model without ever testing it. He prematurely concludes that others won't love him if he reveals his secret. Rather than risk losing their love, he usually decides to keep his secret. This decision then and there sets up either a distancing predisposition or a skeptical, ambivalent view about having close relationships, dynamics that may continue throughout his life.

The sad fact is that the boy's assessment about how receptive his parents will be to his secret is probably accurate. In a homophobic society no parent is going to be made happy or proud upon learning that a son is gay. Rather, the parent hears that the child has an affliction, and the emotional response to the revelation is almost always negative, eliciting sad, painful, angry, or guilty feelings in the parent. Even parents who are lovingly responsive to the son's revelation nonetheless worry about society's acceptance of their child.

What we are suggesting is that, precisely because this is a homophobic culture, a child or adolescent's initial discovery that he is gay is, in and of itself, traumatic. But the discovery is made far more traumatic because he almost always endures it alone. Attachment theory has been called a theory of trauma (Atkinson, 1997) because it examines the intra- and interpersonal consequences of trauma, particularly when the attachment figure is perceived to be unresponsive in helping the individual manage intense emotional experience. Because of the shame they experience in their discovery, most gay youth do not automatically turn to their primary attachment figures for help in managing their emerging homosexuality. They fear that their parents will not be emotionally supportive. The resulting sense of aloneness in managing the trauma has far-reaching implications for how one's emotional life develops from then on.

Diana Fosha (2000) has written about the consequences when the individual cannot turn to significant others for help in managing trauma:

> The individual must choose between preserving the integrity of his attachment ties and that of his affective self experience. Almost invariably, affective experience is sacrificed; access to affects—and with them, all the adaptive resources and richness inherent in experiencing them—becomes deeply compromised. This Faustian bargain (giving away the affective soul in exchange for a measure of security) is effected through defense mechanisms employed against affective experience. (p. 83)

Applied to gay male development, Fosha's ideas suggest that, to preserve his attachment ties, the gay boy learns to repress or ignore his own internal experience in deference to what he believes will be acceptable to others. Not only are his sexual feelings repressed, but also other internal emotions cannot be freely expressed to others. He cannot let others get too close to him for fear of being found out. The end result is that the homosexual boy grows up deprived of a relational context in which his authentic emotional self can emerge and grow. Instead, he becomes increasingly distant from others and emotionally self-reliant. While boys in general are taught to be autonomous and independent from an early age, with the culture valuing and reinforcing these traits more in males than in females (Gilligan, 1982), gay males are forced defensively to become even more separate as a function of their social alienation, whether real or imagined. A gay male often learns it is not safe to turn to others when feeling vulnerable, particularly to other males. Later, in adult life and in a safer context where a gay man might be authentic, real, and vulnerable with another man, he may be totally at a loss for how to behave.

THE DEVELOPMENT OF A FALSE SELF: HOW MANY HOMOSEXUAL BOYS COPE PRIOR TO COMING OUT

Because children are so dependent on their attachment figures for emotional connection, many homosexual males cope by developing, either consciously or unconsciously, a false self they believe will be acceptable to others.[8] They keep the truth to themselves and present a different persona to others. The false self allows the homosexual male to pass as heterosexual, to repress his erotic attraction to other males, to suppress any stereotypically feminine behavioral traits and interests to avoid being called "sissy" and by implication "queer," and to minimize his emotional feelings of attachment to, and dependency on, other males. His true feelings are split off and kept secret from his attachment figures, either parents or close peers. The process of discovering one's homosexuality is rooted in isolation and, unfortunately, continues to grow in a barren, unnourishing soil until he begins to share his discovery with supportive others. Once he begins to share his internal experience and have it accepted, being gay becomes much less traumatic. That is, it is the process of sharing with others that he is homosexual—and having at least some people respond lovingly—that begins to heal the trauma. On the other hand, when significant others respond to his revelation with rejection and judgment, the gay individual can be retraumatized.

Sociologist Erving Goffman (1959) argued that social life requires virtually everyone to have a "public self," and several versions of it, to negotiate situations in everyday life. The public self is the individual's social identity, and may or may not match the individual's private self. Using a dramaturgical metaphor, Goffman believed that the public self was actively and consciously managed and manipulated, based on what the individual "actor" believes the "audience" expects. Gay boys understand that the mainstream culture expects them to be straight, and given the social risks for violating that expectation (taunts of "faggot," "sissy," or "queer"), many gay males consciously develop a public self of heterosexuality, passing as straight. Many become well skilled in im-

---

[8] Winnicott's (1965) use of the term "false self" is a self-portrayal presented by the infant to the mother in order to maintain her attachment. Winnicott theorized that all infants in their profound dependency on the caregiver develop to some degree a "false self" to facilitate getting their basic needs met.

pression management, manipulating the impressions they want others to have of them, in order to avoid the immediate social marginalization that would result if others suspected they were gay. Passing as heterosexual can continue well beyond adolescence, with some gay men marrying and having children.

As Goffman (1963) later noted, compared with other minority groups, passing off a false self in public life is a phenomenon unique to homosexuals. Unlike most other marginalized groups whose ethnic or racial identities cannot be disguised or hidden, a gay man can often choose whether or not to reveal his gayness, making passing an option for him that is not available to other minority groups to avoid discrimination. Although passing may have an adaptive function in that it helps a gay man avoid becoming socially marginalized, it comes at a high cost: *He can never reveal his true core self to the people who matter most to him.* In Bowenian terms, he can never be "an authentic self-in-relation." In Bowlby's terms, if he shows his autonomous self, his attachment figures may very well have nothing more to do with him. So, he hides his true self and passes as someone else. When passing, the homosexual male is living a dual identity, a public self he shows to others and a private self only he knows. He is always on guard never to mix up his worlds. In the mainstream culture where he must watch his pronouns in telling coworkers how he spent the weekend, he may feel, as Andrew Holleran (1978) suggests, like an immigrant in his own country. Like an immigrant, he holds dual citizenship in both mainstream and gay cultures, each with competing values, rituals, and loyalties.

Virtually all gay males go through some period of hiding their sexual orientation from others, and possibly from themselves. The longer such hiding occurs, the longer the man feels shame, the more profound its impact on his ability to form authentic attachments and romantic relationships. *Successful relationships that are deeply intimate require the individuals to reveal and relate to each other's true selves.*

COMING OUT: THE DEVELOPMENT OF A GAY IDENTITY

If the individual proceeds to act on his homosexual orientation by developing a gay identity (and this aspect of homosexuality is indeed a "choice"), he begins the developmental process of "coming out" (Cass, 1979), disclosing to significant others, including his attachment figures, his homosexual orientation. Coming out is ultimately a process of the individual gay man shedding the false self and reclaiming his true identity. It takes courage.

In Bowenian terms, coming out is a moment of real differentiation, defining one's authentic self while risking the relationship. In coming out to those to whom he is most connected, the gay male risks losing those very connections. In a homophobic society it requires enormous agency and individual autonomy for the gay man to reveal to significant others this core truth about himself. In coming out, he puts relationships on the line, as there is always the chance that the other will reject him. Some will. The more significant the person is to the individual, the greater the betrayal, a rejection that qualifies as an "attachment injury" (Johnson, Makinen, & Millikin, 2001). At any point along his developmental journey, a gay man may "foreclose," Cass's term for closing off further development of one's gay identity.

Cass (1979)[9] describes the coming-out process as composed of six developmental stages that can take up to 10 years to complete and may stop without completion at any point. Cass and others assume that the homosexual male begins life, as does everyone else around him, assuming he is heterosexual. He discovers through his fantasies, interests, and experiences that he is attracted to the same sex. The discovery can happen at any point from childhood to late adulthood. Cass assumes that, because of the culture's homophobia, a male is thrown into a state of inner turmoil when he comes to realize that his erotic interests tend to favor males. The state of turmoil and confusion leads to feelings of social alienation, a feeling commonly expressed as "I am the only homosexual in the whole world." In our view, this is where the trauma crystallizes, as the individual usually has no one to help him sort out or understand his feelings. The alienation and turmoil can be so great that some individuals repress or deny their feelings and abort the coming-out process during its incipient stages.

Other homosexual males, seeking ways other than repression or denial to reduce their feelings of alienation, slowly immerse them-

---

[9] The model offered by Cass (1979) is only one model of gay identity development and has its share of critics. But it is a model that is very well known and offers clinicians a number of insights into gay male identity development. For a review of other models, see Reynolds and Hanjorgiris (2000) and Gonsiorek and Rudolph (1991).

selves in the company of other gay persons, identify role models, and begin a period of socialization into a new cultural subgroup that has a stigmatized status. It is at this stage that the individual often feels he has a foot in each world, the gay subculture, where he actively explores his homosexuality, and the mainstream heterosexual culture, where he silently passes as straight. If the coming-out process continues, he grows less ashamed of his homosexuality, begins disclosing it to significant others, and may begin to question or reject mainstream values and institutions. This period of embracing one's homosexuality and the gay community, and being embraced by it, begins to "heal the wounds of external oppression" (Gonsiorek & Rudolph, 1991, p. 174). This period of "gay pride," where homosexuality seems to be the center of the individual's identity, may then evolve into a final stage of identity synthesis, where gay identity becomes only one aspect of the larger self and the person experiences himself as having both similarities to and differences with people of both heterosexual and homosexual orientations.

While the false self does get partially dissolved in the process of coming out, the gay male nonetheless retains a developmental history of holding back, not expressing his true feelings, for fear of social reprisal. Although casting off the false self is psychologically necessary before a gay man can form authentic attachments, many gay men nonetheless carry with them some residual experience of expecting others to be critical, judgmental, and shaming once they reveal their emotions. Gillian Walker (Siegal & Walker, 1999) has put this succinctly:

> Gay men grow up forced to keep everything that is precious about themselves secret, thus confusing what is valued with what is the subject of shame and disavowal. The effects of this growing-up experience are ingrained and longlasting. One man said that, as he revealed something about himself, he would scan his partner for the effect of his revelation. The moment the other person was about to answer, he could feel himself withdrawing, every inch of his body filled with defensiveness and silence, expecting punishment for any act that revealed his authentic experience. It was reflexive—in his muscles. He longed for an authentically honest relationship, but of course his reflexive behavior was not conducive to trust and dialogue, nor was he in fact trained to be comfortable with intimacy. (p. 40)

And, given the reciprocal and complementary nature of relationships, the partner to such a man will of course experience the man's defensiveness and anxiety and undoubtedly have his own reaction to it, either to distance himself if he is uncomfortable encouraging the man's emerging authentic emotions, or to be responsive, patient, and encouraging as the man struggles to be real.

Moreover, as males, gay men have been exposed to the same gender acculturation that all males receive: Men should be strong and not show their feelings. *But, for straight men, male–female relationships are one of the few culturally sanctioned contexts where a man might reveal the full range of his feelings without censure or shame.* In heterosexual romantic relationships it is permissible for a man to let down his guard, show his feelings, and not be judged weak. This is not to say that considerable numbers of straight men do not find intimacy difficult, since adult emotional intimacy violates their earlier years of male gender acculturation. But part of gender acculturation is the male's expectation that females will be more tolerant, accepting, and encouraging of his shortcomings and self-doubts, given their supposedly stronger interest in mutuality and connection.

During adolescence, as they date girls, straight boys form romantic pair bonds that gradually expand their roster of significant attachment figures to include peers (Hazan & Zeifman, 1999). Most straight males get considerable practice in creating relationships during adolescence and young adulthood as they experiment with forming romantic bonds. By contrast, in a homophobic culture most gay adolescents are deprived of this early experimentation with relational romantic experiences with other males. (While gay adolescents may indeed have sex with one another, these incidents often end with the young men feeling shameful, and the sex that occurred does not lead to increased emotional intimacy, as it can in heterosexual pairings.) Gay boys may in fact form close nonsexual relationships with girls, whom they may experience as less critical of their "differentness." But a girl friend is not the same as a girlfriend. For many gay youth, adolescence is a time of extreme isolation. Although clinical research is inconclusive, some studies have shown teenage suicide among gay youth to be disproportionately high (Remafedi, French, Story, Resnick, & Blum, 1998). But it is the curse of loneliness that is far more widespread among gay teenagers, a curse that can afflict them their entire lives.

THE STORY OF DOUG

In our clinical experience as well as that of others (Isay, 1989; Drescher, 1998), gay men frequently report in psychotherapy that they have felt different from others for as long as they can remember. For some, the feeling of being different was present before they could articulate precisely how they were different (Savin-Williams, 1998)—that they are attracted to members of the same sex. For some, the feeling of being different came from within; for others, it originated from how others reacted to them when they engaged in gender-atypical behaviors. Regardless of its origin, the feeling of being different at such an early age can produce a profound rupture between one's self and others.

The first instance when a gay boy realizes that he is different from others can be a quite poignant moment. Doug, 30, a gay man in individual therapy, once described to his therapist how this experience occurred for him. The prompt for recalling the story occurred after a year of therapy at a moment when he was feeling unusually safe with his therapist. The patient was talking about the death of his beloved grandmother, someone whom he felt had loved him deeply. In the middle of his story, as he was conveying his sadness over losing her, without thinking he crossed his legs at his thighs. The change of posture would probably have gone unnoticed by the therapist were it not what Doug did next: He abruptly seemed to "catch himself" and within a split second resituated his legs, laying one ankle atop the opposite knee, taking a more masculine position.

When the therapist inquired about his change in posture, Doug became silent. He appeared deep in thought as he anxiously shuffled his feet. With halting speech and without looking the therapist in the eye, he told him, "Well . ... ever since I was 5 years old, I have been 'acting male.' Just then when I crossed my legs like that . . . well, I guess I forgot the script." The therapist asked him what had happened when he was 5. He told the following story:

> "I grew up in a Midwestern suburban neighborhood and had mostly girls as my friends. The girls taught me to play with dolls and to play 'house,' which I really liked. I thought playing house was the most natural and fun thing in the whole world . . . until kindergarten. When my mother dropped me off for my first day and I spotted

the kitchen play area, I ran over there as fast as I could, where several girls were playing already. Suddenly the boys who saw me began calling me names, 'Look at the girl,' 'Oh, he's a sissy boy,' pointing their fingers, laughing and sneering at me. I didn't understand what I had done to deserve all the ridicule! The teacher quickly came over, scolded me for playing in the girls' play area, and led me to the area where the boys were playing with toy tractors and cars. It was then that I kind of 'got it.' "

This was Doug's first experience of being publicly shamed about an aspect of his sexual identity. Although he did not know then he was homosexual, he experienced an instance of profound humiliation that instilled in him the feeling that he was different from other boys in ways that were strongly disapproved. To cope as a little boy, he quickly learned to adopt, as part of his false self, a masculine demeanor. For him, a masculine demeanor did not come so naturally, although he eventually mastered it. He deliberately studied other boys and imitated the way they walked and moved, much like the character of Albert in *La Cage aux Folles,* who tried—much less successfully than Doug—to imitate John Wayne's lumbering gait. In addition to imitating male gestures, Doug set out to acquire masculine interests such as football, hunting, and dating females. He developed a steady dating but nonsexual relationship with a girl that continued from eighth grade through high school. Once out of high school and no longer under scrutiny by peers and parents, he stopped dating women and began having clandestine sex with men. In college Doug acknowledged to himself that he was gay, but he did not come out to his family or friends. He hated being homosexual and could not imagine his family accepting him. He increasingly became a loner and had no close friends. He continued to keep up his masculine façade, as embodied ultimately in owning and driving a pickup truck in New York City.

Throughout his life, Doug had significant problems with depression, feeling that he did not fit in anywhere. He rarely let anyone get close to him emotionally, preferring to stay isolated and keep his feelings to himself. He continued to have anonymous sex with men. Occasionally these encounters developed into short-lived relationships. They invariably ended when the boyfriend began to push for more emotional intimacy or commitment. Doug was very likable and handsome, and it was no surprise that men would pursue him. But in each budding romance, whenever the boyfriend began to show signs of love and affection, Doug would typically begin pursuing casual sex outside the relationship, rationalizing to himself that he no longer was sexually attracted to his boyfriend.

During the summer that he turned 26, feeling more isolated than ever before, Doug deliberately got himself infected with HIV—that is, he took a share in a beachfront community popular with gay men and proceeded to practice unsafe sex for the entire summer. He consciously reasoned that if he were ill with AIDS he would finally experience connection with others. He envisioned joining AIDS support groups where he would be supported by other men, and he imagined receiving love and sympathy from his parents once they knew he had AIDS. In a visit home to his parents in Minnesota the following winter, he told them he was both gay and HIV-positive. Interestingly, while his parents were loving and sympathetic, he could not internalize their caring and acceptance. Back in New York, when they would call and ask about his health or whom he was dating, he "wouldn't want to talk about it."

Doug's tragic life story derived from feeling that he had never fit in. His pivotal experience in kindergarten where he was simply being himself had taught him that, if he simply was himself, he would be rejected. Although he longed to feel connected with other males, he could never move toward that since he would have to put himself at emotional risk. Moreover, he spent so much time creating and maintaining his false self, he eventually became cut off not only from others but also from his own internal emotional life. His individual psychotherapy focused on his becoming more self-accepting by helping him slowly take in the therapist's accepting and nurturing feelings toward him. The psychotherapeutic relationship became the first accepting relationship he had experienced, a relationship where his "authentic self" could be loved and appreciated. As Jonathan Mohr (1999) has suggested, like many gay men with a high degree of internalized homophobia, Doug had a push-me–pull-me struggle with emotional intimacy, a part of him longing for it but the stronger part terrified of it.

Like many other gay boys exposed to early social humiliation, Doug did not appeal to his parents for comfort after his experience at kindergarten because he was so ashamed. Shame, left unattended, almost always exacerbates, tending to make the individual become ever more isolated and thus filled with greater shame (Wright, 1994). Doug could not easily reach out to his parents because doing so, he imagined, would have provoked their shame of him, making him ultimately feel worse by having the others know. (Consider, though, the outcome if Doug had confided in his parents about what had happened in kindergarten that day. Suppose also they had been empathic, supported Doug's interests even though they are what society regards as feminine, talked with him about how children can sometimes be cruel, and possibly worked with him on how to express his own individual interests in a world that may not always value them.) Instead, Doug developed an internal working model that his authentic self was unlovable by others. Never able to take in nurturing relations from other men because he so hated his own true self, he turned more and more inward and got increasingly depressed. He could not imagine, or experience, a male figure being responsive and available to him, even when potential boyfriends were. His emotional avoidance of men was so strong that it wasn't until his psychotherapy that he began to have a corrective experience, as he began to trust his male therapist.

OTHER MEN'S STORIES

As a representative of a gay man's development, Doug is neither typical nor unique. Some gay boys have more alienating and isolating experiences than Doug, particularly those boys who cannot suppress their feminine behavior and interests and do not develop a false persona. These boys may either lack the skills to manage the impressions they make on others, or have the skills but choose on principle not to present a false image of themselves. Other gay boys have less socially alienating experiences, especially gay boys who develop masculine behavior and interests more naturally than Doug. Masculinity per se becomes part of the core self rather than a façade. But more masculine gay boys must still develop a heterosexual façade to get through childhood and adolescence. The point is, again, that gay boys can hardly ever be real and authentic.

In our clinical experience, a small minority of a younger generation of American-raised gay men claims not to have experienced initial confusion when they discovered they were attracted to men. But, while these men were more accepting of their gayness from the outset, they all had strong doubts that others would be so accepting and devised ways for managing their homosexuality. For example, one man, Jack, reported that, once he realized he was attracted to men, he thereafter feigned being straight until he was no longer dependent on his parents. He said:

> "It was all just an act. I always knew who I was and I had no particular problem with being gay. But I knew everyone else would. So I dated girls, played sports well enough not to cause any suspicion, and acted like I was straight. I was always very clear who I was, and I knew what I was doing was just an act. Maybe this is why I became a professional actor: I've been in a role much of my life! But once I had some money of my own, I came out to my family, and it was curtains on that performance."

Once Jack did come out to his family, upon graduation from college when he was no longer financially dependent on them, they accepted his homosexuality with minimal distress, and he continues to enjoy a satisfactory relationship with them.

A similar individual, Luke, took the same approach in dealing with his homosexuality but got different results. Although he always had been strongly attracted to men and was clear in his own mind that he was gay, he nevertheless dated and had sexual relations with women, played competitive sports, and passed as straight. He was gregarious and had a large network of straight friends, but he longed to be in an intimate relationship with another man. At age 30, he decided to come out to his parents. The outcome was disastrous. Having until then viewed Luke as their golden prince, a son who had amassed considerable academic, professional, and social achievements, his parents could not tolerate his homosexuality. Although Luke steadfastly refused, his parents pushed him to enter reparative or conversion therapy (Nicolosi, 1991), a form of psychotherapy that attempts to alter homosexual orientation, even though evidence indicates such efforts are seldom successful and actually cause harm to patients (Shidlo, Shroeder, & Drescher, 2002). Luke has yet to have a steady boyfriend or more than a couple of dates with any man. He has mostly anonymous casual sex. This delay in developmental dating experience is not atypical of gay men we see in either individual or couple therapy in our practices. Luke's parents still maintain a relationship with him, but talk about his homosexuality is almost completely avoided. If the topic does come up, his parents typically start blaming him for his "choice." His siblings will chime in by accusing him of "ruining Christmas" the year that he came out and "destroying" their mother for the next year (who cried endlessly over the fate of her son). For Luke, his own realization that he was gay may not have been traumatic, but coming out to his parents and siblings certainly was.

These examples illustrate how gay males, in order to survive, learn to live in emotional isolation out of fear, either real or imagined, that others won't be supportive or empathic. Some develop adaptive skills favoring individual autonomy, throwing their energies into academics, sports, or music. Others learn to soothe themselves in less constructive ways, through substance abuse or compulsive sex.

SUMMARY

Although most gay males arrive at young adulthood longing for intimate relationships with other men, they often find close emotional connections with other men at best unfamiliar and at worst impossibly difficult. Early experiences particularly with the father and male peers make the gay boy feel rejected, different from others, and alone. To defend against his shame and to defend against his needs for dependency, attachment, and connection, he places exaggerated importance on his own self-reliance and emotional autonomy during childhood and adolescence. Denied relationships with other males where he can authentically connect (i.e., reveal his true self while deeply connecting with the other) but still needing some connection with others, he may develop a false self, a façade of strong individuality and separateness, particularly when interacting with other males. Because his own internalized homophobia makes him feel shameful about his desire for emotional and sexual intimacy with other males, he is reticent to seek nurturance and emotional sustenance from them. While the false self allows him to have some relational experience, so long as others do not know a vital fact about him—that he is gay—authentic and deep emotional connection is rare. His deeper relationships are often with women instead, and women may be some of the first persons to whom he comes out. Rarely does he turn to men for emotional support, and, given the choice, he would rather rely on himself than on another man.

Yet, as a human being, the gay male craves connection. Despite his well-honed autonomy and separateness, he yearns to connect emotionally with another man. As he begins to form adult romantic relationships with men, some tendency to be emotionally withholding and to be distrustful may remain from the years of practice he has had in keeping his own counsel and not making himself vulnerable to other men. Moreover, the cultural prescriptions about the level of emotional intimacy permissible between males, which all males cannot help but internalize, contribute to keeping him feeling disconnected from his male partner. The autonomy and separateness he developed as defensive coping mechanisms in his earlier years, and which served him well then, are no longer so adaptive. At this point, his individuality, autonomy, and separateness are overly developed and now interfere with his desire to connect and relate intimately to another man. Deeper connection is remote and foreign to him.

Couple therapy can be viewed as an opportunity to alter closeness–distance dynamics and attachment styles.[10] Once intimacy issues emerge in the couple's treatment, the men's defenses around strong individuality and emotional self-reliance will need to be confronted, challenged, and broken down in order to allow new, more relational, resources to emerge. As we will see, our model challenges male couples actively in session to break up rigid patterns of closeness–distance cycles, pushing each man to expand his previous range of functioning, which for gay men is often toward developing a capacity for greater connectedness. Although our techniques are from structural family therapy, our theory is informed by Bowen and Bowlby in that we push the couple to become "authentic selves in relation" and to develop secure attachments to each other. This is hard work for many male couples, since they, like everyone else, arrive at adulthood with relatively fixed levels of differentiation and particular attachment styles, which for gay men is a style often too oriented toward maintaining a sense of separate autonomy and a

---

[10] Susan Johnson's (1999; Johnson et al., 2001) emotionally focused couple therapy is perhaps the first model of couple treatment to be based on attachment theory. Some of her clinical work focuses on situations in which a vulnerable member of a couple feels betrayed by the other, creating an experience so devastating that it lingers on, contaminating subsequent interactions between them. Johnson calls the incident an "attachment injury" (2001) and structures the therapy sessions in order to repair the injury actively in session. She helps the couple reengage emotionally, specifically coaching the "betrayer" to develop more empathic feelings for the partner's experience. Although our clinical interventions are technically different from those of Johnson et al., we agree that couple therapy is a special venue to alter old attachment dynamics.

skepticism about getting too close. Therapy pushes them to jumpstart their growth process anew. For gay male couples, this is particularly difficult work since they have had difficulty with authenticity from the days of early childhood. As we have seen, gay males in their early development—because they feel they must hide the secret of their homosexuality—have often been deprived of authenticity in their relationships with significant others. In their youth the true self could not be revealed—or so it was feared—else their connection with their primary caregivers might be completely severed. It is the fear of losing the connection if they reveal their gayness that makes the experience of homosexuality so traumatic.

While couple therapists need to be sensitive to these early developmental experiences of gay men, therapists must not let their understanding and empathy for such experiences put chains around them. As structural therapists, we believe it is necessary for therapists to challenge the couple to get out of their ruts and to cut new grooves. We unbalance and introduce novelty in an attempt "to loosen the knots" (Gerson, 2001). Couple treatment, in other words, is a different time and place than childhood and adolescence. The gay man needs to have an experience in therapy where he can form a secure attachment to his partner without surrendering himself. Moreover, following Minuchin's faith in the resourcefulness of individuals, we make the assumption that the resources to do this are already present—that is, that men in general, and gay men in particular, are not inherently deficient in relational skills. They simply haven't practiced them enough with other men. The skills are dormant, awaiting activation by the structural therapist.

CHAPTER THREE

An Overview
of Structural Family Therapy

In this chapter we will present an overview of a structural model of couple therapy that is applicable when working with all family systems and present a heterosexual couple to illustrate the generic model so we can begin to compare both similarities and differences that exist between gay male couples and heterosexual couples. Our model is adapted from Salvador Minuchin's structural family therapy (Minuchin et al., 1996; Minuchin & Nichols, 1993; Minuchin & Fishman, 1981; Minuchin, 1974) and consists of three stages. As we describe the generic model, we will illustrate the three stages with a case study that is intended to teach the family therapist (1) how to join with a couple, (2) how to create enactments so that the therapist can observe a couple's complementary roles that maintain their presenting problem, and (3) how to unbalance and expand a couple's preferred style of relating to each other.

Recently Trudy and Jed, a young heterosexual couple, came into one of our offices. The expectant wife, Trudy, was very anxious and sat on the edge of her chair, appearing to be ready to burst at the seams as she waited to speak. Her husband, Jed, who had been 10 minutes late, tiptoed into the session and slipped into the other chair. He looked the therapist over skeptically and nodded hello. He appeared to be there against his better judgment and slouched down in the chair as if he wanted to disappear. Before the therapist could ask why they had come in for treatment, the wife blurted out, "I feel like I'm being held prisoner by my husband!"

The following day, a male couple, Hal and Bill, arrived in the same waiting room 15 minutes before their scheduled appointment. As the therapist was preparing for the afternoon, he walked through the waiting room to make a cup of tea. One of the two men, Hal, expensively but casually dressed, was slumped in a chair glaring at his partner. If looks could kill, he had sufficient ammunition. Bill, his partner, dressed in a Brooks Brothers suit and highly shined cordovans, was busily absorbed in making notes on a document. The therapist introduced himself and asked them to come into his office. Before they were seated, Hal tore into Bill, accusing him of bringing his law practice along to the couple's session. "I want out of this relationship," he announced.

Neither of these examples is an unusual scenario of the first minutes of an initial session, and both illustrate the linear explanation common to most couples as they present themselves for treatment. The implicit message in these two vignettes is "Fix him and our problems will be solved!" We as structural family therapists view this linear attribution, which focuses on the problematic behavior of one of the individuals in the relationship, as significant but overly simplistic. Structural family therapy has at its core a belief in the interconnectedness of all human behavior. Behavior never exists in isolation but is organized and influenced by, and in response to, our relationship with others. We all construct patterns of behavior that are organized by our relationships and interactions with others. These patterns, if they become rigid and inflexible, are sources of stress for a couple. And, they frequently are a narrow definition of our complexity and resourcefulness as human beings in relationship to one another.

We first focus on identifying these patterns of co-constructed behavior and then encourage a couple to expand their repertoire of behaviors to discover new ways of relating, utilizing inherent but dormant resources of the individuals in the system. Ema Genijovich (1994), a family therapist and founding member of The Minuchin Center for the Family, refers to this dynamic of identifying the untapped resources as the therapist's search for "hidden treasures." While acknowledging the seriousness of a couple or family's presenting problem, a therapist simultaneously begins to formulate hypotheses about the circular interpersonal behaviors that maintain the patterns. As systemic clinicians, we are always looking to expand the presenting problem to include behaviors that both partners are doing that maintain their "stuckness."

Specifically, rather than accept one individual's story as the sole explanation of a couple's unhappiness, we introduce during the early stages of treatment alternative stories that connect their behaviors to one another. We call this expansion of the problem that uses the language of complementarity, reframing (Minuchin & Fishman, 1981). Simply stated, rather than thinking that a couple's problem resides in one person, we begin to reformulate the presenting problem as one that is maintained by circular causality (Bateson, 1979), the interpersonal behaviors of people in a family or by a family's interactions with larger systems. How we do that is the focus of this introduction to family therapy.

The three-stage model that we will first introduce and then illustrate with clinical cases throughout this volume is a map to help guide the therapist through treatment with couples. The model is not intended to be used linearly. The more experienced the therapist is with the model, the more she may simultaneously weave various stages together.

THE BASIC MODEL

Joining,[1] a necessary stage of any treatment, is something that most therapists do automatically, even if they are just beginning to do clinical work with family systems. However, the focus in this initial stage of couple treatment differs from the initial stage of individual treatment. Individual treatment usually focuses on the early history of the problem and how the individual came to create his belief system that informs his individual patterns of behavior. In contrast, couple treatment focuses initially not on the early developmental history of the individuals in the system but on the formative history of the relationship and under what circumstances the presenting problem appears in the relationship. When we focus on the individual's past in the clinical cases presented here, it is to better understand the current dynamics of the couple.

We all have a valance or predisposition for certain behaviors that generally complement the behaviors of the partners we choose in life (Bowen, 1978). However, when these complementary behaviors be-

---

[1] See Haley's (1987) Chapter 1 for further information on conducting the initial family interview.

come rigid, couples get caught in patterns of behavior that are either dissatisfying or inhibit their potential for growth. When a couple comes to a therapist for family treatment, generally one partner has been labeled as "the patient" and the nonpatient partner in the relationship has called the therapist to make an appointment for the errant party to be cured or fixed.

Another way in which systemic treatment differs from individual treatment is that, with the exception of mandated cases, clients in individual treatment generally come in voluntarily, expressing a desire to change their behavioral, emotional, or cognitive patterns. In family treatment, one or more members of the system are often reluctant to be in the therapist's office and may be present only under duress. Consequently, a therapist must spend more time in joining with family systems to engage the reluctant members.

When a couple comes for family therapy, generally one (if not both) of the partners is dissatisfied with the limited, inflexible patterns of behavior that they have created. What's typical in our clinical experience as illustrated with the straight and gay couples referred to at the beginning of this chapter is the difference between a straight and a gay couple's initial attempts to solve the problem. The explicit message from Trudy in the first case is "I've brought him to be fixed." But with the gay couple, although one partner locates the problem in the other's behavior, Hal's solution is to avoid the conflict and disconnect from Bill (i.e., "I want out of this relationship").

Although a generalization, these drastically different responses to a crisis in the relationship highlights one of the ways in which joining with straight and gay couples differs. Straight couples usually have large, extended networks of family members and friends, and larger systems such as civil law, that support and give them an incentive to maintain their marriage. Gay couples that come for family treatment are often isolated from their families and mistrustful of larger systems (of which the mental health system is a part) where they have experienced rejection and shame. As described in Chapter 2, a gay man's mistrust of attachment figures and significant others often extends to his partner. For many men, the learned pattern of response in the presence of conflict is to disconnect to protect oneself. The joining phase for family therapists must incorporate an understanding of these different responses to conflict so that a therapist can earn the trust of a couple and engage them in treatment. Joining with gay couples is often a longer process, which we will focus on in the next chapter.

JOINING

During the earliest stage of treatment it is essential that the therapist form a therapeutic alliance with the new clients. The overt task in this initial stage is for the therapist to hear each client's version of the presenting problem and to take a history of when and how the problem began. Besides gathering essential clinical information that enables the therapist to make hypotheses about what are the interpersonal behaviors that maintain a couple's problem, equally relevant, the couple and the therapist are getting to know one another.

Do the clients feel they can trust the therapist? Do they feel safe in her office? Will the therapist pathologize or shame them (a particularly sensitive issue for gay couples or any other minority group)? No therapeutic interventions can occur until a couple feels that a therapist is there to help them and that they can entrust their relationship to the treatment process. A family therapist eventually will be asking a couple to reveal their very private patterns of behavior and then will be encouraging them to risk changing those cherished behaviors. Therefore, in this early stage of treatment, it is essential that a couple experience a therapist as both professional and respectful of them. It is not necessary, nor even desirable, for them to feel relaxed in the office. A certain degree of tension is therapeutic if a couple is going to be motivated to change their behavior.

Therapists often err in thinking a couple must be enamored of them. During the early stages of treatment, in fact, this attitude is counterproductive to therapy. A therapist can wait until termination occurs to experience their gratitude. Another common error for family therapists eager for a couple to experience their expertise is to challenge a couple's preferred style of relating before acquiring their trust.

A therapeutic alliance must exist that communicates both respect and professionalism. A therapist needs to convey that he will structure the session so that both parties are heard and no one will be disrespected during the session. Language is important in this process. A therapist's selective use of a couple's language helps to convey empathy and understanding. During early stages of treatment, though, therapists should avoid use of the vernacular or slang. This is particularly true in working with older couples. Youth can work as an advantage for a young therapist as she initially takes a subordinate role in the session. Acknowledging differences conveys a therapist's respect for a couple and enables the couple to feel empowered in the process. As the first session begins, the therapist can create structure by asking a few simple questions.

Once the couple is inside the therapist's office and introductions are completed, the therapist can ask how they were referred for treatment and reiterate the presenting problem if previously communicated by one partner during the initial telephone contact. The purpose here is for the therapist to communicate that she is not in collusion with any one partner. These first few moments are also giving the couple and the therapist a transition or bridge from the everyday world that they have just left to the unique culture of the therapy session. The rules of behavior will be altered in this time and place, and the therapist needs to convey the significance of this transition while simultaneously making the couple feel welcomed.

We find it helpful to videotape couple sessions for learning purposes. Other than live supervision from behind a one-way mirror, viewing and discussing videotaped sessions is the most effective method for a family therapist to obtain supervision. Viewing taped sessions also gives a therapist opportunities to understand to what extent she may have lost objectivity and has become inducted into the couple's dynamics. A therapist may also show excerpts of the videotaped session to a couple in order to ask their help in understanding their dynamics. If taping, a therapist will need to explain to a couple that sessions are recorded for training purposes and that she would like their signed consent to do so during their treatment. A sample consent form is illustrated in Figure 3.1. Generally speaking, unless a therapist is working with a high-profile couple, most couples have less reticence about being videotaped than new therapists have about requesting permission.

A therapist may also need to reiterate to a couple the length of the session. Many family therapists do 60- to 90-minute sessions, as opposed to the 50-minute analytic hour, and a couple may need to be reminded of the time boundaries that exist for a session.

Once a therapist has obtained permission to videotape and has acclimated the couple to the therapy, it's generally advisable to ask them several questions. The therapist's role at this early stage of treatment is to help focus and organize the session. Couples and families will present themselves for treatment with a lifetime of information that the therapist must help them sort in order to focus on the relevant issues for treatment—otherwise, both they and the therapist can feel overwhelmed. "What brings you into treatment?" or "How can I help you?" are two

Therapist's Name

Therapist's Address

CONSENT FOR VIDEOTAPE RECORDING OF SESSIONS

We the undersigned consent to the videotaping of our therapy sessions with [*thera-pist's name*]. We release [*therapist's name*] from any liability in connection with the use of such materials.

It is understood that the videotape recording will be used for training purposes only. We waive all rights that we may have to any claims or payment.

Clients' Signatures:

_____

_____

Date: _____

FIGURE 3.1. Sample consent form.

simple questions that are often helpful to focus the session. As in the clinical examples used at the beginning of this chapter, usually the partner who has brought the couple into treatment will speak at this time. A therapist should allow sufficient time for him to speak but not allow any one partner to dominate the session. After a therapist has gotten a sense of what the problem is from that person's point of view, it is often helpful to summarize what that partner has said. This conveys to the person that he has been heard and helps the therapist to make a transition. The therapist then needs to encourage the other partner to tell why he or she has come for treatment. The therapist might make the transition by saying, "I want to hear more from you, but it's also important that I hear what changes your partner would like to see happen to improve the relationship. Tell me, why are you here?"

Again, the use of language is important. "What would you like to see change to *improve* the relationship?" implies that the therapist believes that a couple has the capacity both to change and improve their relationship. Conversely, asking "What's wrong with your relationship?" encourages them to engage in nonconstructive criticism of each other. Also, giving each partner an opportunity to voice his concerns for the relationship conveys to him that the therapist is interested in hearing both points of view. No one person is the holder of the ultimate truth. As the therapist continues to join with the couple, he begins to gather information about the history of the couple's relationship.

After each partner has told the therapist what each of them would like to see changed in order to improve their relationship, it's important for the therapist to acknowledge to them that their presenting problem has been heard. At this point, the therapist might summarize what the second partner has said in order to communicate to him that he has been heard and to make another transition. The therapist will be returning to the presenting problem, but it's important that she gets to know both partners in the context of their whole relationship. The therapist might say exactly that to them: "We'll return to this problem that's causing you both a lot of pain, but first I would like to get to know you as a couple." Alternatively, the experienced family therapist might choose to encourage a couple to engage in an interactional pattern of behavior, an enactment. Using as an example Trudy and Jed, the therapist said, "Your wife says you're holding her hostage. Can you talk to her about that?" However, for clinicians new to this model, we encourage therapists initially to be more joined with a couple before staging an enactment. A therapist can make a mental note of their apparent interactional style and continue the joining process as she takes their history.

As mentioned earlier, the history a therapist takes at this early stage of treatment focuses on the time a couple has spent together. Clinicians trained in individual psychotherapy are inclined to focus on an individual's history even when treating a family. If in the early stages of treatment a therapist focuses on the origins of an individual's behavior, she risks meeting resistance when she reframes the presenting problem as symptomatic of a couple's interactional patterns. In the beginning as the therapist joins with the couple, he is educating them to the culture of systems thinking. Central to the practice of this therapy is the belief that families and couples construct one another, activating limited complementary behaviors (Minuchin, 1974). Each individual's past is relevant only insofar as it contributes to and maintains a couple's current dynamics.

When we use the term "complementarity," we are referring to a dynamic that exists in all systems regardless of their size. Couples develop interactional patterns of behavior that provide for mutual support and create interdependence. The family therapist automatically knows that if one partner in a couple is overfunctioning then the other partner must be underfunctioning. If one partner is performing "the parental role" in a relationship, then his partner will be in the complementary role of "the child."

Using a food analogy, it might be helpful for a therapist to think of the concept of complementary behaviors as "the pizza theory" of human behavior—rather than thinking of individuals as "onions" that need to be peeled in order to get to the core of their psychopathology. George Simon, another founding member of The Minuchin Center, often uses Jorge Colapinto's metaphor of people as "pizzas" interacting with one another. Each person is like a pizza—consisting of slices of character traits and strengths that can be activated by other people's complementary behaviors and that are interacted with in specific contexts. As with Felix and Oscar in Neil Simon's play *The Odd Couple*, a partner who is prone to being neat needs by definition to interact with a partner whom he can pick up after—otherwise, "the neat freak" is unemployed.

Following the initial honeymoon period in a couple's relationship, patterns of behavior that initially attracted the partners to each other may become rigid and even sources of stress in the relationship. When a couple comes in for treatment, it is the therapist's job to create the conditions for change during the session with the couple. The belief inherent in this treatment model is that people have the inner resources and strength to develop more complex and rewarding relationships than they are currently experiencing.

As the therapist takes the history of the early stages of the couple's relationship, she begins to formulate hypotheses about the limited complementary roles that they have accessed in their interconnectedness with each other. The therapist is already beginning to redefine the couple's behaviors as their limited responses to each other and to larger systems (i.e., the interactions between a couple and the majority culture; the majority culture's attitudes toward race, ethnicity, socioeconomic status, and sexual orientation). A therapist may even at this early stage of treatment make her hypotheses explicit to a couple.

To the underfunctioning partner, a therapist might say, "So when you feel unneeded at home, you become more involved with your work?" And to the overfunctioning partner she might connect that behavior pattern by saying, "And it sounds like when he gets too involved with his work, you feel abandoned and resentful. You feel over-burdened with home responsibilities. Have you ever been successful at getting him more interested in you and the home?" In this way the therapist simultaneously begins to connect the partners' circular patterns of behavior, while also creating a therapeutic culture that acknowledges and supports interdependency and complementarity.

JOINING WITH TRUDY AND JED: TWO INDIVIDUALS BECOMING A COUPLE

When Trudy and Jed presented for treatment, they were in their late 30s and expecting their first child. They came from similar backgrounds, each having grown up in a second-generation Swedish American family with similar economic status and religious values. The presenting problem was that Trudy was miserable in the couple's new home in the suburbs. She felt bored and isolated in the suburbs, preferring the urban environment of New York City, where she was born and raised. She felt that Jed was unreasonable and unwilling to attempt to understand her unhappiness. In their first session Trudy expressed her unhappiness to the therapist while her husband sat tight-lipped and red-faced. Trudy had a forum in the therapy room, and she seemed to believe that, if she could recruit an ally in the therapist, she would succeed in convincing her husband to move back to the city. In contrast, Jed sat fuming, red in the face, refusing to engage in any dialogue.

Trudy accused Jed of being rigid and inflexible. Eventually, as the therapist began to hear from "the patient," a reportedly tyrannical husband, the story became more complex as he expressed his fears that his wife was more connected to her siblings than to him. However, this complexity did not emerge in the first session. The therapist erred as he experienced a pull to support Trudy. His oversight in not hearing the husband's fears of abandonment resulted in the husband initially refusing to come to the next session. In order to repair this and more fully join with him, the therapist had to call the husband and invite him to the next session. The therapist also apologized in the next session, admitting that he had erred in not hearing both stories. Only after the therapist joined further with Jed, and heard his side, could he connect their behaviors to interpersonal responses to each other, to the possible pulls they were experiencing from their families of origin, and to the stresses of preparing for their first child.

Both individuals were college-educated and had mid-level management jobs in investment banking. Prior to treatment, they had maintained individual checking accounts and had never considered merging their finances. Married for 7 years, the couple appeared to never have negotiated any division of labor in their home. Both Trudy and Jed were highly competent in their careers, and yet none of Trudy's competence appeared to have translated to the making of a home. When the therapist queried them about how they made family decisions, Trudy said that she had always acquiesced and allowed Jed to make the major decisions.

For instance, after they had moved to their new house in the suburbs, they had purchased a second car for her use. She had wanted a station wagon in anticipation of children, but Jed said they should get a sedan. Although she did not agree, she reported stifling her feelings to avoid any argument. Similarly, when they took vacations, Trudy reported doing what Jed wanted in order to avoid disagreement. However, in anticipation of a soon-to-be-born child and the discontinuance of her career to become a full-time mom, Trudy said she was feeling panic at the thoughts of living full-time in the suburbs, separated from her siblings and parents in the city. As she described in session this panic to her husband, Jed gradually turned bright red and glared at her and continued to refuse to engage in any dialogue.

Although neither partner was physically or verbally abusive, Trudy retreated when she encountered her husband's obstinate style. Initially, it appeared to the therapist that the way that she had expressed her displeasure with him was to avoid any participation in the running of the household. Eventually, now in her second trimester, she began spending first days and then nights in her parents' apartment in the city. As the therapist encouraged her to talk in session to her husband about her loneliness in the suburbs, when met with his silence she turned and attempted to engage the therapist in a coalition against him. "Am I unreasonable?" she asked. "Why can't he see my perspective?" Trudy's attempts to triangulate the therapist, the therapist came to believe, reflected the basic dynamic in how the two partners avoided disagreements at home. The couple was not comfortable engaging in a dialogue or in challenging each other. With a baby about to be born, Trudy was attempting to change the unwritten rules of their marriage that gave Jed the power to be the sole decision maker. Jed was trying his best to cope with the conflict by avoiding the issues and continuing as if nothing had changed. Trudy increasingly turned to her parents and siblings for support, just as in session she turned to the therapist.

Jed appeared baffled by Trudy's misery, stating that she should be grateful for their new home and a standard of living that neither of their parents had been able to achieve. Trudy countered that she had never lived in the suburbs and found them boring and isolating. If Jed would only accommodate her wishes, she said nervously, all would be well in their marriage.

Caught in an alliance with Trudy and in danger of losing Jed, the therapist at this point in treatment made a mental map of the couple's relationship. If he stayed with their argument, he would continue to be drawn into the tug-of-war in which they were engaged. Now was the time to think developmentally.

Where were they in their life cycle as a couple? Although about to become a threesome with the arrival of a baby, they seemed to be caught up as a couple in an early developmental stage of creating a new family identity. Trudy seemed to be struggling with differentiation from her family of origin, and the therapist wondered if this couple had ever transferred their primary loyalty to each other. Trudy's split loyalties were more obvious, but the therapist wondered if Jed's commitment to living in the suburbs might be based upon their home's proximity to his family. This thinking created a bind for the therapist, as the couple appeared then to be caught in a symmetrical power struggle. Symmetrical power struggles are not only rare but difficult for a therapist to unbalance. He decided to encourage more enactments so that he could observe their dance and identify the complementary roles that maintained their stuckness.

FOCUSING ON A COUPLE'S STRENGTHS

As the therapist continues to join with a couple, he begins to expand their presenting problem from one of linear causality to the possibility that the problem is maintained by complementary behaviors both in the context of the couple's system and in their interactions with larger systems. Simultaneously he begins to identify inherent strengths in the relationship as he asks history-taking questions to make inquiries into how the couple met. "Do you remember your first date?" "Tell me when you knew that you had fallen in love with your partner. What characteristics were you initially drawn to in him?" "Have you an anniversary date that you celebrate together?"

Questions that focus on rituals creating a family system are important for all couples but particularly salient for gay couples. Because gay relationships are only just beginning to be socially and legally recognized in the United States, gay couples have not traditionally had either the legal or community support that might help them create an identity as a family. Consequently, many gay couples benefit from creating commitment ceremonies that help them establish an identity separate from their biological and adult extended family of friends. Questions that focus on anniversaries and commitment ceremonies are also therapeutic for a gay couple, as the question immediately signals to them that the therapist regards them as a family. We will expand upon this theme in Chapter 4.

Additionally it is important to get the early history of the relationship to ascertain under what circumstances the couple came to be together, whether they had a long courtship or whether they even have made a commitment to each other and to their relationship. The therapist will thereby begin to get an idea of whether the couple has a firm foundation on which to build their relationship. Couples who report an early period of idealized love, as did Trudy and Jed, often have that as a common bond to use in recommitting to each other during stressful times. Another matter of importance to discover is what their decision-making style has been like as a couple.

As the therapist continues taking the history of the couple's relationship, she is making structural hypotheses of how they have co-constructed their interactions, and she is getting to know each of them within the context of their relationship. During this stage of treatment the therapist is working closely or proximally with a family to understand them and the world that they live in. (We use the word "family" interchangeably with the word "couple" in this volume. We think of couples as families regardless of whether or not they have children. Childless couples have a complex network of friends and biological relatives that they interact with. Gay couples often create adult families of choice, a collection of nonbiologically related people who interact in roles similar to those in traditional heterosexual families.) (Green & Mitchell, 2002).

A COUPLE'S INTERACTIONS WITH LARGER SYSTEMS

A couple never exists in isolation and is always shaped not only by the partners' interactions with each other but also by their interactions with larger systems. If the couple is part of a marginalized minority, it is important for the therapist to ascertain whether they have joined together in alliance against the discriminating majority culture or, conversely, have turned perhaps some of their latent anger on each other? If theirs is an immigrant family, what have been the challenges of moving to a culture in which they are a minority? What are the effects of their being separated from their biological family abroad? Have they been able to create an adult extended family in their new country? If the partners are from different ethnic groups, how do the cultures of their two clans complement each other? Do the partners have similar religious or spiritual philosophies? Do their families and friends support their relationship?

It is important for a therapist to begin to understand how a couple interacts with and is organized by their interactions with larger systems. Although in the United States we do not often speak of class, access to power is influenced not only by socioeconomic status but also by gender, race, ethnicity, and sexual orientation. For instance, for a family of color presenting with issues of substance abuse, in addition to inquiries about drug treatment, it would be important for the therapist to ascertain how the drug usage might be a means of self-medication for depression related to experiences of racism by the majority culture. Or if a couple is an immigrant family and they have no biological relatives in this country, what stresses has the experience of being uprooted from family and friends brought into their marriage? If they are bilingual, have they learned yet to think in the new language, and if so how has that affected them? How, conversely, has their immigrant status further *isolated* them?

If these history-taking questions sound political, they are meant to be. Therapists are often working with and advocating for families that are isolated because of who they are. This isolation creates stress on a family that is destructive to the stability of the couple's relationship. A therapist needs to be comfortable in exploring how a family experiences marginalization and to learn what adaptations the couple has had to make.

It is also important for the therapist to be aware of the life cycles of the family (Carter & McGoldrick, 1989, 1998). The tasks for a new couple just beginning to get to know each other and fall in love are considerably different from the tasks of a couple in the seventh year of their relationship who are also considering having children. Whereas a new couple is learning to respond to each other's needs, a couple about to have a baby must expand their system to accommodate the needs of a dependent infant. The focus of the relationship for a couple with a new infant shifts dramatically, and the transition can create stress for a couple. Or, as in the case of Trudy and Jed, a couple may be struggling simultaneously to create an identity as a family separate from their families of origin as they also prepare to accommodate the needs of their first child.

While a therapist should never underestimate the knowledge obtainable from her own life and educational experiences, she also must rely upon each family to teach her about their unique experience. If she doesn't know about their experience—and it is wisest to assume that at the outset—she can simply ask them to explain. Oddly enough, the families that can be the most challenging for a therapist to work with are those whose experiences are most similar to her own family's. It's all too easy to assume that one knows one's own and their issues best. In such cases the therapist often misses the obvious systemic conflicts that she might see more readily in a family different from her own culture.

All of the foregoing issues are relevant in working with both heterosexual and gay couples. Issues of marginalization and discrimination become more complex when working with gay couples. For instance, two gay white males in a committed relationship in our society will have many of the unearned socioeconomic privileges that their gender and race afford them but they may be entirely bereft of biological and extended family support systems. A heterosexual family of color in our society feels the socioeconomic effects of being a marginalized minority but may experience strength from the support of fellow church members and a large extended family. The absence of family and community support can be just as significant in undermining the stability of the family as socioeconomic discrimination.

STRUCTURAL MAPPING

During the early stages of treatment the structural therapist maps (Minuchin, 1974) the family's dynamics to further understand how they have created and maintained the complementary patterns of behavior in their relationship. The map is a visual schema that represents how a therapist experiences a couple, and it should denote the multidimensional complexity of family systems. Initially the therapist is looking at boundaries, hierarchy, emotional style, and accommodation to ascertain how the couple respond to each other's needs. When a therapist thinks about boundaries (Minuchin & Fishman, 1981; Nichols & Schwartz, 1998), she is looking to see if a family has successfully created an identity that separates them from other systems. Boundaries can be rigid, permeable, or nonexistent, and each of these characteristics has ramifications for the functioning of the family system.

Ideally, family boundaries need to be permeable but clear. While creating an identity for the family, people need to be able to enter and exit the system to function in the world. Families with rigid boundaries often are overly controlling of its members, as people sometimes have trouble creating an identity that allows for both an "I" and a "we." Families with rigid boundaries frequently have difficulty in hearing their individual voices. People in such systems often talk in "we" phrases, and it's difficult for a therapist to understand an individual's needs in this system. Members may resort to conflict in an attempt to individuate and be heard. A strength of families with rigid boundaries is that they can be highly responsive to one another's needs and often have prodigious internal resources for responding in a family crisis.

Families with nonexistent boundaries, characteristic of poor families involved with multiple social service agencies, have trouble maintaining an identity as important decisions affecting the family are made by outside social service agencies (Minuchin, Colapinto, & Minuchin, 1998). The dilution of a family's decision-making process (Colapinto, 1995) that occurs for families involved with multiple social agencies is problematic, as outside agencies become "the experts" in the family, disempowering the family in a complementary dynamic that labels the family as "the incompetents." The process of decision making, essential to the family's identity, becomes the responsibility of social agencies. A family becomes disengaged and disconnected as family conflicts are resolved by outside "experts." Middle-class families, as we will discover in the case of Trudy and Jed, can also have nonexisting boundaries when the partners have not shifted their primary loyalties from their biological families to their newly created family.

Ideally, members should be able to enter and exit a family system and still maintain an identity with the family that is appropriate for any given stage of development. Hierarchy with an executive subsystem needs to exist to ensure the well-being of a family. For instance, infants are dependent on the family for all of their needs, but teenagers' developmental task is to begin to individuate while still staying connected to the family as the teenagers gradually transition into adulthood. Families often present themselves for treatment when they experience crises in making important transitions from one stage of their developmental life cycle to another (Carter & McGoldrick, 1989). For example, when a couple decides to have a child, as in the case of Trudy and Jed, one or both partners can experience stress as they expand their dyadic relationship to accommodate the needs of a third entity. Often, one partner feels unneeded and unwanted as the other partner takes up the role of the primary caretaker of the infant. Couples need to be able to negotiate and maintain their identity as a couple as they simultaneously divide up child-rearing responsibilities to function as a family. These tasks are the same for gay as well as heterosexual couples.

Gay couples struggle with the same tasks of expanding the dyadic relationship to include and meet the needs of a new member, or to incorporate children into a blended family, as do heterosexual couples. Additional stresses exist for gay families due to the isolation and prejudice they may experience from the majority culture. Often they experience intense pressure to be "perfect parents" in response to the majority culture's skepticism about their rights to child-rearing privileges (Martin, 1993). A couple may inadvertently attribute these stresses to differences in parenting style when they present for treatment. It is necessary for a family therapist to be knowledgeable about the effects of minority status on gay couples and to help a couple expand their presenting problem to include any stresses related to external prejudice.

One of the many stresses that bring families into treatment today is the challenge that couples experience as the traditional family is redefined. Women are experiencing greater, though not equal, earning power and greater access to careers that historically have been closed to them. Blended families—where one or both partners have been previously in a committed relationship and bring children from that relationship into a new family—are common. The distribution of responsibilities in a family must continually be redefined as families expand and contract and cope with the new roles of women in society.

Fluidity of roles is most typical of gay couples, for whom there is an absence of traditional role models (Green et al., 1996). Although the freedom to negotiate roles can be liberating for gay couples, as they are able to create relationships that are not confined to stereotypical roles, gender acculturation conflicts and the avoidance of dependency roles are often sources of stress for many men. Two men in a committed relationship are faced with the added dilemma of what it means to be a follower of—or dependent upon—another man. Frequently gay men enter relationships in which complementary roles have been largely predetermined by age differences or by educational or financial disparities. The partners must gradually renegotiate these roles over time if the relationship is to grow.

For reasons previously discussed in Chapter 2, gay men often use couple treatment to repair and heal prior traumatic relationships that impede intimacy with each other. The trauma that they have experienced from the majority culture (as with many other minorities) is either turned inward or into the relationship rather than the two using each other as a resource to buffer prejudice (Allport, 1958). Interestingly, as women prosper in their quest for greater equality, heterosexual couples and gay couples experience greater similarities. "Who's on top?" becomes a question that all couples must struggle with. Can both partners take turns as leader and follower as they take advantage of each other's strengths?

Mapping is one way for the therapist to visualize the couple's dynamics with each other and their relationship to larger systems, and guides the therapist in helping a couple discover new roles. During the early stages, when two individuals come together to form a new system, the couple's first task is to create an identity as a family separate from their family of origin and any extended adult family of friends. All couples must go through a process analogous to separation and individuation in adolescence. The task for a couple is to create an identity that says to the world, "We are a family with an identity separate from our biological and adult families of choice."

Culture and the unique idiosyncratic characteristics of each family come into play here. If one partner is a Latin American Jew and the other partner a first-generation Irish American Catholic, two very different cultures are coming together to create a new system. When we think of Latin and Jewish family values, we often expect to find an emphasis placed on closeness and family connectedness. We can either characterize this closeness as pathological and label it "enmeshment," or we can reframe high family dependency as a strength, particularly in times of crisis when a family's members must collaborate with one another.

In contrast, many Irish American families are often experienced as being disconnected, with strong values being placed on individuality and self-reliance. The tendency to disconnect is an emotional style that may have evolved, probably enabling individuals to survive the Irish Diaspora of the 19th century, when millions of Irish immigrants were forced to leave their homeland, or perish from starvation. The propensity to disconnect may interact with and reinforce a cultural bias that devalues and avoids interpersonal conflict. Two individuals from dissimilar cultures will have to negotiate with and accommodate each other as they create their own "third" family identity. Such challenges in creating a separate identity as a "we" also exist for couples who are from similar cultural backgrounds.

As a couple seeks to create an identity, the second developmental task they encounter is accommodation (Nichols & Minuchin, 1999). It's important for the therapist to ascertain how a couple accommodates each other's needs on a day-to-day basis. If the couple lives together, have they successfully created a division of labor in their household? Whether or not they live together, it's important for the therapist to ascertain how much time they spend together. In two-career families, couples frequently don't spend enough time with each other to create their own culture. When they come together, they may experience tension as they make the emotional transition from the workplace to their home.

A good question that will help a therapist ascertain much useful information is, "Tell me what a typical weekday is like for the two of you, from the time you get up until you go to bed." This question helps a therapist to ascertain what the couple's lifestyle is like. Do they know each other, or are they strangers occupying the same bed? Do they spend sufficient time with each other to have developed a language of "we-ness," or are they always focused on their individual needs? Many couples, especially two-career couples, need to schedule time together to give their marriage, or relationship, the priority it deserves. Asking a couple what they enjoy doing together and how frequently will give the therapist some insight into how much time they spend together and how many interests they share in common.

MAPPING TRUDY AND JED'S RELATIONSHIP

A tentative map of Trudy and Jed's relationship illustrates the key dynamics of their family system. History taking revealed that, when treatment began, Trudy was spending most of her free time at her parents' home. Though married for several years, the couple appeared to never have negotiated a division of labor. Jed did most of the house-related chores. He was overfunctioning in their system, and his wife was in the complementary role of underfunctioning. The couple had made no preparation for the imminent birth of their baby. They were unable to talk to each other about their dissatisfaction with their current living arrangements for fear that conflict would result in a permanent separation. Trudy chose to spend much of her free time with her family rather than confront her husband with her dissatisfaction.

Figure 3.2 illustrates one hypothesis of how Trudy and Jed had constructed their relationship. If accurate, the map will serve as a guide for the therapist in his work with the couple. In order for Trudy to connect with Jed, the couple will need to create an alliance with each other. The therapist will now need to encourage the couple to interact to ascertain what behaviors maintain their mutually inflexible roles.

If the therapist's schedule permits, sessions that are scheduled for an hour and a half will provide her with the time needed to do this work. This is particularly true for the first session, when the therapist must gather a great deal of information and still give the couple some sense of therapeutic change and hope before the session ends. Because this model of family therapy is a short-term treatment based upon

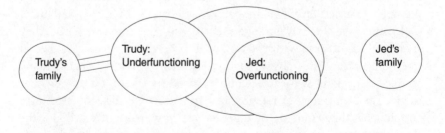

FIGURE 3.2. Structural map for Trudy and Jed.

change that occurs in session, the therapist ideally wants the couple to experience some growth or expansion of their style within each session. Minimally, a couple needs to experience in session the circular dance that they do that maintains their being stuck in predictable patterns of behavior. We advise that therapists give themselves, at a minimum, 60-minute sessions in order to allow for this to happen.

ENACTMENTS: THE THERAPIST SETS THE STAGE FOR A COUPLE'S INTERACTIONS

Until now, the task for the therapist has been to focus on joining with the family while simultaneously taking a history of the system. Unless a therapeutic alliance has been established with the couple, they will not trust the therapist to enter their system and challenge them to relate in new ways. Taking a history enables them to get to know the therapist and for the therapist to get to know the family as he begins to formulate hypotheses about them. Up to this point in the session, the therapist has been central and proximal to the couple. It is now time for him to assume a less prominent role so that he can observe their dynamics as a couple.

If a couple is seated together, which they generally will be if there is a sofa in the office, it is now time for the therapist to ask one of the partners to move to a chair so that they can face each other. (Generally speaking, sofas are best used for breaks when the therapist wants a nap. A sofa, in forcing partners to sit close together, encourages intimacy and diminishes possible challenging interactions between them.) As the therapist rearranges the seating, couples who have never been in treatment will often look at the therapist in bewilderment. They expect her to do the work and to be the holder of all knowledge in the session. By asking the couple to begin to work with each other, the therapist is communicating to them that they need to find the answers *with each other.*

Many couples, particularly those who are estranged or disengaged, will initially resist talking with each other. Couples who are emotionally shy with each other will need to be gently nudged. The therapist needs to encourage the partners to interact with each other, and eventually they'll understand that she won't settle for less.

The only exception to this rule arises when working with high-conflict couples. If the therapist feels the need to diminish affect in the session, she should remain central and direct each partner to talk to her only. Other than separating a couple, this is the best way to lower affect and the potential for conflict in a session. However, these cases are rare, and a therapist will generally need a couple to interact in order to ascertain what their interactional style is like. She should encourage each person to speak for himself.

Enactments (Minuchin & Fishman, 1981; Nichols, 1997; Nichols & Fellenberg, 2000) provide an in-session experience for the therapist to observe how the couple relate to each other. Families usually present themselves for treatment at transition stages in their life cycle that have precipitated crises in their interconnectedness. A family system experiences stress as the transition challenges the couple's homeostasis. As the therapist encourages the couple to relate to each other rather than direct their comments to her, the underlying construction of their relationship will begin to become apparent. The interactions that the therapist observes in session offer an enactment, or microcosm of behavior, of how a couple interact with each other outside of treatment. The enactment provides a snapshot of their relationship.

For couples who are disengaged and reticent to express feelings with each other, the therapist may want to encourage more affect in the session. This is also true for couples that are depressed and where the affect is flat. With these couples, the therapist will want them to choose a controversial topic. For disengaged partners, such as Trudy and Jed, the therapist said, "When do you think your wife became more interested in her family than you? Tell her directly and I'll listen."

If the therapist desires to focus on the strengths of a couple's relationship, which is often initially important for couples that are highly stressed, she might ask one partner to tell the other what is was that first attracted him. "Can you tell your partner what characteristics initially attracted you to her?" If the partner persists in talking directly to the therapist, she can simply say, "I'll listen, please tell your partner." The purpose of the enactment is for the therapist to observe how the couple communicates, problem solves, and negotiates differences. Once the therapist has sufficient observed data, she can feel more secure in her hypotheses. She can then begin to unbalance and challenge the couple to experiment with new behaviors.

ENACTMENTS WITH TRUDY AND JED

When Trudy and Jed entered treatment, though married for several years, they interacted as though they were still single and dating each other. Both had careers that they enjoyed and found financially rewarding. Jed had grown up in a home in the suburbs and enjoyed taking care of the yard. He was a good cook and had assumed the tasks of shopping and cooking. Trudy was underfunctioning, possibly as a way, however ineffective, to express her resentment toward Jed's unwillingness to listen to her. Like many overfunctioning partners, Jed resented Trudy's lack of participation in the daily chores of making a home but was unaware of how he had discouraged her participation. Jed had never expressed his disappointment in this inequitable arrangement with his wife. He expected that she should be able to read his mind and know what he wanted. She was both amazed and relieved to hear him begin to talk in session about his frustration and sadness.

Initially conversing together was difficult for both of them. Trudy flooded with emotion and Jed withdrew, which only increased Trudy's anxiety that he would not respond to her. Eventually, as Jed started to talk with her as an equal, Trudy stopped running and started to listen to him.

Slowly, with encouragement from the therapist, Jed began to talk to his wife. He initially said he felt her plan to move to the city was a conspiracy to live closer to her siblings. For the first time in treatment, he became vocal as he expressed frustration and anger at Trudy's desire to be back in her old neighborhood. As he addressed his wife in the enactment, Jed's communication style was revealed. The problem was he didn't just talk with her, he barked his thoughts out. He grew red in the face and blurted out, "You just want to be closer to your family! I won't live near them." The therapist, not wanting to discourage Jed from talking just as he had found his voice, chose for the time being to ignore Jed's abrupt style of communicating with Trudy. Trudy looked stymied and turned to the therapist for help. The therapist, supporting Jed, asked Trudy if she knew why her husband was so opposed to living closer to her family.

Trudy was speechless.

During the course of taking their history, Jed had briefly mentioned spending all major holidays with Trudy's family. She reported growing up in a family that she characterized as matriarchal. She said that her mother dominated her father and made all the major decisions. Even though Trudy's siblings were married with children, her mother continued to be "switchboard central" for all of her children's lives. Jed said he grew up in a family where both parents shared in the decision-making process.

The therapist wondered aloud if his harsh tones with his wife might be an expression of his fear that they would re-create her parent's marital dynamics in their own relationship? The therapist continued to support Jed's becoming more active in the sessions as he simultaneously challenged Jed's behavior. He asked Jed to experiment with his style of communication. The therapist wanted to see if Jed could talk to Trudy so that she could hear him and so she felt encouraged to respond, to come closer. "Jed, I think your wife may be anxious about becoming a first-time mother. Can you help her?"

Still red in the face, Jed stammered as he attempted to speak to her in a softer voice that would encourage her to respond. Jed then talked to Trudy about his fear that she was going to become like her mother. Although it had not been stated, the therapist speculated that Jed was anxious about becoming a new dad and feared that he would lose both his voice and his wife, once they became parents.

Like many men, gay or straight, Jed confused disagreement with hostility. He went into a "fight or flight" mode when his wife challenged him. His emotional style was to avoid disagreement or to issue ultimatums to Trudy if she pushed him too hard. Trudy's style was to initially engage and then to disconnect when she met Jed's resistance. At one point she retreated and moved back into her family's home for support when she and Jed experienced a stalemate in this major transition in their marriage.

The first goal of their treatment—a task that until now they had avoided—was for them to create an identity as a couple separate from their families. Could they establish a boundary to reinforce their identity as a family? Concurrently Trudy and Jed needed to experiment with new collaborative behaviors to prepare for the anticipated addition to their family. In working with this family in the process of formation, the therapist helped Trudy and Jed to focus on their mutual needs as he encouraged them to develop a more equitable style of decision making.

Now that Jed was engaged in the treatment, the therapist shifted the focus of the sessions to whether the partners would be successful in creating a home for their soon-to-arrive child? He asked Jed to talk with

his wife. Could he invite her back to their new home? Initially Jed resisted talking to her. Reverting back to the early stages of treatment,
Trudy preferred to talk with the therapist and Jed preferred to abstain
from talking. Such resistance is common when couples are more comfortable avoiding conflict and have not developed a common language.
The therapist simply kept reiterating to Jed, "Talk with your wife."

Jed again took his preferred authoritarian position: "Either you
move back in or the marriage is over." The therapist interrupted this
pattern of communication, using as leverage Jed's obvious happiness
over his anticipation of becoming a father. During earlier sessions, talking about the upcoming birth of their child was the only time that Jed
and Trudy had sounded like a couple. They were in agreement that they
wanted the best home for their child. "Jed, I wonder if you're going to
get Trudy to move back in time for the baby's birth by making that kind
of ultimatum," the therapist inquired skeptically. "Trudy, can you tell
your husband whether that invitation for you to return worked for
you."

The therapist, securely joined with Jed, was now able to safely support Trudy's voice at this point in treatment. Trudy was able to tell Jed
that she felt unseen and dismissed when he made ultimatums, as he had
just done. She expressed her fear that he was not interested in her happiness or well-being as an expectant mother. Jed softened his harsh style
of communication as for the first time he became tearful talking to her
about his loneliness. "We should be living together, and I want you
home when the baby comes," he said.

UNBALANCING: TRUDY AND JED
DISCOVER NEW WAYS OF RELATING

During the unbalancing stage of treatment (Minuchin & Fishman,
1981), the therapist, in a sense, holds up a mirror to the couple and
says, "This is what I observe as I watch you interact." Generally, the
therapist will focus on the complementary behaviors that she has observed and challenge the couple to expand their style of relatedness. For
a couple such as Trudy and Jed that presents as one partner overfunctioning and the other underfunctioning, the therapist said to the
overfunctioning husband, "You must be exhausted doing all this work.
Can you imagine yourself giving up some of the responsibility?" Jed re-

sponded and the therapist directed him to talk with his wife. Or to the underfunctioning wife, he said, "When did you retire from the relationship? Have you always felt expendable?" As Trudy began to respond, the therapist directed her to talk with Jed.

Once a therapist has identified the complementary roles that sustain a couple's dance, he wants to empower the couple to challenge each other to explore novelty and new ways of relating with each other—to discover new steps.

With a structural map and his observation of their negotiating style, the therapist was freer to intervene in a way that began to introduce novelty into the couple's system. Jed needed to find a way to lower his wife's anxiety and invite her to come closer to him.

As Trudy and Jed began to listen to each other, their work as a couple became more collaborative. They initially focused on what they would like to see changed in their marriage. As they both were still working during the daytime, the therapist inquired whether Trudy might want to reconsider Jed's now softened invitation to move back into their home. "Meeting once a week to talk about your future as parents doesn't seem to give you sufficient time for planning," the therapist observed. As a transition to moving back to their home, the therapist encouraged Trudy and Jed to spend more time together. One evening a week they began doing something they mutually enjoyed, usually a concert or dinner in the city. On the weekends, they also began to spend a block of time together doing something pleasurable. If they couldn't mutually agree on some activity, the therapist encouraged them to take turns following each other's lead. During this stage of treatment, the therapist created a context for the couple to experiment with new ways of relating to each other, one that encouraged greater interdependency.

As the couple gradually became more comfortable in closer proximity to each other, the therapist became more intermediate in his relationship to them. He encouraged more interactions between them and resisted Trudy's attempts to triangulate him in their marital discussions. "Talk to your husband," the therapist constantly repeated. During the next 2 to 3 weeks, the couple began to work in session on how they would divide up chores in their home. In one session, Jed expressed his frustration to Trudy about her lack of participation in the day-to-day activities of running their home. When they had moved to the suburbs, not only did he do all the yard work but also he did all the shopping and preparing of meals. He resented this inequity in the household and

Trudy's lack of involvement. In a collaborative response she agreed to take over the cooking responsibilities, and they began to do the food shopping together on the weekends. This negotiating style and ability to compromise for the good of the marriage was new for them. The therapist encouraged them to use sessions to experiment with this new behavior and even to plan dinner menus, for example, during session time.

When the therapist discovered that Trudy and Jed had not created a nursery, he spontaneously demonstrated his amazement. "No nursery has been created for your baby that is due in 3 months!" he exclaimed. "Do you plan to create one as Trudy goes into labor?" Choosing furniture and paint for their home became a joint project but one that Trudy took the lead in by choosing the styles and colors. Trudy and Jed began to bridge their independent worlds, and these simple joint tasks helped them to create their own family identity. The skills they used in dividing up chores, purchasing furniture, and painting the nursery helped them to build confidence that they could collaborate.

The couple's treatment also created a forum for them to negotiate how and where they would spend family holidays. Jed for the first time began to voice his unhappiness with their current arrangement. In the end, they were able to accommodate each other's desires—Trudy's desire to spend time with her siblings and Jed's desire to make a home. For instance, on Mother's Day, rather than go to her parents' home, which they had traditionally done, Trudy agreed to her husband's plan to take her out for a special dinner to honor her new status. Jed became more agreeable to spending time with his in-laws as his wife became more participatory in the making of their home. Instead of permitting her mother to make holiday family decisions for them, Trudy began to set limits with her mother. She began, at first hesitantly, to tell her mother that she would first confer with her husband before agreeing to any invitations. The couple also began spending more time in their new home, and invited both families over for a traditional Sunday dinner.

At this stage of treatment, once Trudy had returned home, the couple decided that it was time to discontinue treatment. Trudy and Jed had taken the initial steps in creating an identity as a family and in negotiating a more satisfying relationship, and their first child was about to be born. Trudy had not entirely lost her distaste for the suburbs. But, with her restored self-confidence and experience that Jed would listen to her, combined with Jed's willingness to be more open with his feelings,

Trudy made a compromise. She decided to go along with Jed's desire to stay in the suburbs for now as they began to decorate their home and create a nursery. The therapist encouraged them to come back for a follow-up visit after the baby arrived.

Transitions, such as the birth of a child, are events in the life cycle of a family that can be stressful. A family therapist can help couples to normalize these periods and create an environment conducive to exploring novel approaches and new initiatives. We don't want a family to feel that they have failed if they experience the need to return to treatment. It's not uncommon for a couple to return for sessions at some transition point in their lives if the initial treatment has been helpful.

The discovery and internalization of new ways of relating that are more satisfying for a family requires reinforcement and repetition until the behaviors become routine for them. In systemic treatment, the middle and end stages of therapy are often used to reinforce and consolidate a family's new behaviors.

In the case of Trudy and Jed, the therapist was not clear at the end of treatment whether they had consolidated the new roles that they had discovered during treatment. The unbalancing of old behaviors had occurred early in their treatment. Though the presenting problem initially had been Trudy's fear that she was being "held hostage" in the suburbs, as treatment progressed, the couple discovered they were both hostages. They neither had created mutual trust for agreement nor had they demonstrated a willingness to make compromises in their marriage. As treatment ended, they both experienced a more satisfying relationship that prioritized their marriage (see Figure 3.3).

The task of learning how to accommodate the needs of the new system challenges couples differently depending upon the culture that each of the partners grew up in. For families such as Jed's that placed a high value on independence and avoidance of conflict, and Trudy's that valued matriarchy, becoming a "we" in a new relationship challenged their individual values. Prioritizing the relationship over their individual needs felt as though the self or "I" might be subsumed.

The emphasis that many couples place on individual needs is a value reinforced by the culture or society in which one lives. The popularity of literature in the United States on the subject of codependency attests to an underlying fear of becoming "pathologically" dependent upon anyone or anything.

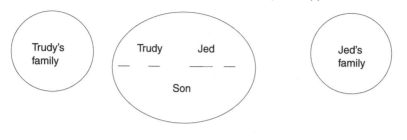

FIGURE 3.3. New map for Trudy and Jed.

REVIEW OF TRUDY AND JED'S TREATMENT

Trudy and Jed needed to create a system whose emotional style would enable them to feel safe as they learned to resolve their differences. Their style of communication, revealed early in treatment, was to avoid emotional conflict and disconnect rather than to negotiate with each other. Historically, their mutual problems went unresolved, and numerous disconnects had occurred in Trudy's family from one generation to another as grudges were maintained by the family's emotional style. Whether to avoid conflict or attempting to interrupt cross-generational patterns, Trudy and Jed created a marriage in which Jed made all the major decisions. Trudy had concurred with this arrangement. When Trudy became pregnant, she began to question their style of decision making. For the first time in their marriage, she began to challenge her husband. Jed became overwhelmed and frightened by her new voice, and in response he closed down. Faced with Jed's wall of silence and feeling unsupported, Trudy moved back home to her biological family that valued matriarchy while Jed proceeded to live alone. When they discovered that their differences were not going to miraculously be resolved, they came to family counseling, which provided them with a safe neutral forum to openly disagree for the first time since becoming a couple.

Though the couple presented with a linear presenting problem (i.e., Trudy brought Jed in to be fixed), the therapist used the language of complementarity to educate the couple as to how they had co-constructed their marriage. The therapist initially questioned how they had created a marriage with an overfunctioning husband. Challenging the couple's preferred style of avoidance, the therapist raised the possibility that it was easy for Trudy to go home to her mother, as she had no clear role in her home with Jed. In an effort to avoid conflict, they had constructed a marriage that left Trudy "unemployed." Could Trudy get Jed to give her some of his household tasks? Could Jed ask Trudy to take over some of his responsibilities? Their complementary behavior featuring an underfunctioning Trudy could only exist so long as Jed overfunctioned in the relationship. The therapist said to the husband, "You're angry with Trudy because you feel like you're overworking at home. How have you managed to create a wife who feels that she's extraneous?"

When it became clear through enactments that Jed gave Trudy the silent treatment when he was angry with her, the therapist kept the focus on the couple's system and increased the intensity: "Trudy, how is it that you have created a husband who is frightened to challenge you?" Later, the therapist focused on the anticipatory anxiety that Trudy was experiencing as she prepared to have her baby. He challenged Jed to be more supportive as Trudy took the lead in preparing a nursery for their son and normalized Trudy's need for her mother's support after delivery.

The language of complementarity proved instructive for the couple. However, they often resisted the idea that they were collectively responsible for the dynamics of their marriage. The therapist's use of repetition of these complementary themes created an intensity in treatment and encouraged them to experiment with new behaviors. If one partner did not get the concept of co-construction, the other partner often would. The therapist then solicited him or her to be his co-therapist for that moment as he supported that partner to elicit new behavior from the other. "Jed," he said, "your wife's accomplished at work. How have you managed to make her incompetent at home?"

A lesson that the therapist learned in treating this couple was to avoid siding with one partner too early, as the other partner will become alienated. If the therapist joins with one partner to unbalance the system, he must make sure that he is first sufficiently joined with the other partner. The therapist does not need to be entirely equitable in creating challenges for the individuals in the system, but the family should experience the therapist as not favoring one partner over the other. For the treatment to be effective, the therapist needs to convey that he respects and values each individual in the system.

Once Trudy and Jed began to experience their new identity as a family, they discovered the resources to teach each other how to accommodate the other's needs. Jed learned how to invite his wife to participate more in home activities. As he became less authoritarian and more communicative, Trudy was willing to be more responsive to his needs. Trudy's responsiveness reinforced Jed's being more supportive of her new status as a mother. They both began to experience pride in their new roles as parents. The therapist was able to use their new status as parents to create a forum for them to learn to collaborate with each other. Interestingly, in a follow-up session after their son was born, Jed told the therapist how Trudy took the lead in making many parenting decisions. He praised her competency as they showed the therapist pictures of their son. The work that they had done as a couple gave them the strength and skills to minimize the stress of having a new baby in their family.

A COUPLE'S A COUPLE AND . . .

What is often ignored by family therapists new to working with gay couples is the importance of a network of friends and family to support and stabilize families. Trudy and Jed had a long courtship as they got to know each other's family and friends. When they decided to formalize their union, they had the legal right to have a ceremony that established them as a family within their social network and in the courts of law. These rituals and legal documents helped to bind and hold them together as a couple. Only with the existence of antidiscrimination laws have gay couples dared to come out and participate in ceremonies to honor their unions. As of this writing, federal benefits are denied to gay and lesbian partners and, with the exception of Vermont, no state legally recognizes committed gay and lesbian partners.[2] The dual tasks of creating an identity and learning to accommodate each other's needs are essential for all couples but become problematic for gay couples since they lack societal and legal support systems. We will describe interventions that specifically address these needs for gay couples in the next three chapters.

---

[2] The Federal Defense of Marriage Act (1996) precludes federal recognition of same-sex marriages. The state of Vermont passed legislation in 1999 that grants equal rights to gay and lesbian couples through the Civil Unions Act in that state only.

CHAPTER FOUR

Joining with Male Couples

In the preceding chapter we outlined the generic model of structural couple therapy. We demonstrated the model using a heterosexual couple to illustrate the three stages of treatment. In this chapter we will elaborate in greater detail our way of working with male couples so that the reader will have a clearer sense of what is different in working with this group, as compared to straight couples. Whatever the couple's sexual orientation and presenting problems, what remains constant is the three-stage structural model. In this and the succeeding two chapters, we will introduce male couples that we've worked with, whom we will use to illustrate the model as we track their progress through treatment.

TASKS OF JOINING

Joining is a critical initial stage of the therapeutic encounter. Unless a couple trusts a therapist and has some degree of confidence that they can benefit from intervention, they will either drop out of treatment prematurely or resist any challenge by the therapist to change their behavior. A couple's pull toward homeostasis is powerful, and their resistance can defeat the most experienced therapist. Structural family therapy is a short-term treatment, and the therapy moves along quickly. The therapist must take charge of each session, which during the joining phase helps to inspire trust from the couple.

The axiom of having to earn the clients' trust and respect, which is essential during the first phase of treatment, is even truer when working with stigmatized populations such as male couples. Just as with the straight couple, a gay couple entering treatment is in crisis and seeking relief. But for a gay couple entering treatment there are two major differences. One is that they often come in defensively, fearing the therapist will judge them, uncertain whether their relationship is valued and worth saving. Second, few gay men we see in our practices have had the experience of working through differences with significant male others. Many gay men have the impulse to flee at the first sign of conflict, and there are few social or legal structures in place to support men working to repair their relationship.

As we noted in Chapter 2, gay men prior to entering treatment have internalized a message from early developmental experiences that they are less than or inferior to the heterosexual majority. Shame-inducing experiences become internalized as low self-esteem, and many gay men have developed a "false self" in childhood that is integrated into their personality by adulthood. These traumatic experiences can be expressed in adulthood in one of two preferred styles of relating:

1. The gay adult may avoid intimate relationships with other men for fear of repeating earlier negative experiences. The attitude of "I refuse to be mocked again" creates obstacles in building an intimate relationship with another man.
2. The gay man may experience and express his need for affection and intimacy with another man as being so precious that he has a desire to merge with his beloved. In this scenario, the partners risk losing their individuality.

Either dynamic, disengagement or enmeshment, is problematic in long-term relationships.

Gay bars, parks, and clubs where it is safe to approach another gay man have frequently been the key gathering places in a gay man's initial socialization and sexual experiences. Same-sex relationships are often kept secret from family, straight friends, and work colleagues. Little societal support exists for a male couple, and relationships are easily dissolved in this milieu. The socialization process for men, regardless of sexual orientation, traditionally rewards independent, stoic behavior. "Boys don't cry" is axiomatic in U.S. culture. Additionally, men in general are socialized to either dominate the other or avoid conflict, often being acculturated to believe that compromising is the same as "los-

ing"—and losers are sissies. Given the secretiveness of many gay relationships and a society that privileges male stoicism and independence,
many gay couples choose to go their separate ways when confronted
with seemingly irreconcilable differences.

It's interesting to note that many of these "irreconcilable differences" are not dissimilar to the boundary-making and accommodation
issues of heterosexual couples. However, gay couples, bereft of role
models, often lack the experience to contextualize their struggles for
creating relationships. This atmosphere of instability and dearth of positive socialization experiences are two significant respects in which a
male couple's experience differs from that of their straight counterpart.

Although heterosexual couples can come to therapy for help in
separating, the majority of such couples are committed to resolving
their differences. Separation and divorce are the last, not first, options.
In the face of conflict, gay couples often feel that separation is the first
option of choice. Creating a therapy that honors and values gay relationships is an essential first step in helping the male couple solidify
their relationship.

FORMING THE THERAPEUTIC ALLIANCE

How is the foregoing knowledge helpful to the therapist, either gay or
straight, who is working with same-sex couples? When a gay couple
presents themselves for treatment, their antennae will be tuned for any
suggestion of homophobia. Nancy Boyd-Franklin (1989) refers to this
guardedness on the part of Black clients as "a healthy paranoia," the clients' adaptation to an unsafe world. It is essential for the therapist to be
prepared for this dynamic and communicate to the couple that they are
in a safe environment.

Creating a nonhomophobic environment begins with the initial
telephone call. In contrast to the initial contact with a heterosexual couple, the gay man calling to make an appointment will commonly ask if
the therapist is gay. We advise that the therapist answer this question directly. In family therapy the therapist is not interested in encouraging
the client's transference, so she becomes a neutral object on which a client can project his psychological process. Structural family therapists
are more interested in creating interactions between the couple so that
the therapist can explore the ways that each partner has contributed to

creating the dynamics of their relationship. If a therapist is gay, there is usually no further discussion once that information is disclosed. If she isn't, she can say just that. During a couple's initial session, she will have the opportunity to demonstrate her respect for gay couples, and the couple can then make the decision whether they want to work with a straight therapist. In our experience, many gay couples initially are more accepting of straight female therapists and more guarded with straight or gay male therapists. Exploration of the meaning of the therapist's sexual orientation or other questions can usually be deferred to the initial session.

Often a couple will also ask about the therapist's fee, participation in managed-care programs, and theoretical orientation. The first two questions can be easily answered, with discussion of the appropriateness of a sliding-scale fee normally deferred to the first session. The last question, regarding the therapist's theoretical orientation, usually reflects the couple's anxiety about the therapeutic encounter. The therapist should answer the question as succinctly as possible: "I'm a social worker (psychologist, psychiatrist) and I have advanced training in family therapy." We usually recommend that a therapist inform a couple that she would like to meet with them for a one- or two-session consultation, so she can ascertain if she can help them, and so a couple can decide if they feel comfortable working with the therapist. The time length of each consultation should also be stated. Again, we recommend that each session be a minimum of 1 hour and, if possible for the initial consultation, 1½ hours. The extra half-hour gives the therapist time to take an initial history and to begin to experience how the couple interact with each other.

Therapists often overlook the importance of having a welcoming waiting room and office that communicates openness to working with gay couples. The therapist can have gay-affirmative literature in the waiting room such as *In the Family*, a magazine that focuses on alternative families. For instance, one straight therapist who is an amateur photographer has pictures of the local Gay Pride Day parade on his office wall. Literature in the waiting room that is supportive of gay relationships or that promotes gay-affirmative community activities and organizations makes a positive statement to gay clients. If the therapist uses an intake form, the marital status portion of the form should have language that reflects gay inclusiveness (see Figure 4.1).

Initially a therapist can help put a couple at ease by asking a few

Name_____ Telephone number _____

Address_____ City_____ State _____ ZIP _____

Date of birth_____

Status: Single _____ Domestic partner _____ Married _____

　　　　　Separated _____ Widowed _____ Divorced _____

　　If partnered or married, person's name _____

　　How long together?_____

Partnered or married previously?_____ If yes, how long?_____

Do you have children?_____　　　No. of girls _____ Ages _____

　　　　　　　　　　　　　　　No. of boys_____ Ages _____

Education: Highest grade or degree _____

Mother: Living _____　　　　　If deceased, when? _____

Father: Living _____　　　　　If deceased, when? _____

Siblings? _____　No. of sisters _____　　No. of brothers _____

Any deceased? _____

Type of work you are doing now _____

Name and address of employer _____

Telephone no. _____ Length of time in position _____

Have you had any illnesses? _____

Hospitalizations?_____ If yes, why and how long? _____

Medications_____

　　Reasons for meds _____

Previous counseling? _____ If yes, how long? _____

If yes, what type and with whom? _____

When did you discontinue? _____ Why? _____

FIGURE 4.1. Intake form.

simple questions as they make the transition into the office. "Was it difficult getting here? Did you encounter a lot of traffic? The elevators are archaic in this building. Did you think you'd have to walk up?" Humor can often help to create a bridge. These questions may sound like idle chatter, but they help ease a couple from one world into the therapeutic environ of a couple's session.

If a couple has filled out an intake form, a therapist will need a few minutes to look at their responses. Alternatively, many clinicians gather this information as part of the joining process. We find it most helpful to have the couple write down certain basic information on the form (i.e., telephone numbers, addresses, relevant medical history) so that we do not need to be writing during the session. We find that a lot of writing during the session can be distracting, and during the early sessions it may act to distance the therapist from the clients. The therapist will also want to orient the couple to her office. If she will be recording the sessions and has not discussed that with them, this is a good time to explain why the therapist records sessions and to obtain the couple's signed permission (see Figure 3.1). "I like to record my sessions because it gives me an opportunity to further explore our sessions and understand how I might be more helpful to you." Or if a therapist is in supervision, " I record my sessions because I consult with a senior colleague when I feel stuck in a session or when I need a neutral informed opinion. And unless we agree otherwise, I erase the tapes as soon as I have had an opportunity to look at them." A therapist can also say that the videotapes can be used for playback in a session with the couple so that they can help the therapist understand what dynamic is being created between them. Usually a new family therapist is more anxious about asking for permission to tape than the couple is about being taped. If the therapist is clear and matter-of-fact about the reasons for taping, most couples will readily give permission. Those who don't give permission initially may be persuaded of the utility of taping during later sessions.

THE PRESENTING PROBLEM

Once the therapist has oriented the couple to the office, the next task is to ask each partner to state why he is seeking treatment. A therapist needs to be in charge in this stage of treatment and create safety in the initial encounter by structuring and leading the session. She might ask a couple, "What brings you in *as a couple*?" or "How can I be helpful to you *as a couple*?" The language is simple but the message is complex. The therapist is communicating both that she recognizes the partners *as a couple* and that she wants initially to get to know them *as a couple*. In asking the question, she has not addressed a specific person but rather she has asked them as a system why they have come into treatment.

Questions about each man's individual history of gay identity development are also important, as those experiences will impact on the men's
relationship. We advise though that questions focusing on an individual's development be deferred initially until the therapist has a better
appreciation of the couple's presenting problem.

This initial encounter is important for all couples but especially so
for gay couples, as the therapist's office may be one of the few places in
the gay couple's lives where they are seen and acknowledged as a family.
This acknowledgment alone can be therapeutic for a couple. A therapist
is also beginning to educate a couple to the unique culture of systemic
therapy by focusing on their collective history. The therapist wants to
communicate to the couple that she wants to hear each partner's voice
and not let one person speak for the system.

When a couple comes into treatment, they are in crisis, and each
partner should have the space to express his frustration and anger. Similar to the heterosexual couple, Trudy and Jed, presented in the preceding chapter, gay couples usually present with overly simplistic explanations of their problem that identify one partner as "the patient," such as:
"My partner is always working and when he is home he watches television. He's not interested in me anymore." Or, "I'd like to have an open
relationship. Tom doesn't want one. He's so inhibited." "Jim stopped going to NA [Narcotics Anonymous] meetings and I'm anxious that he's
using drugs again. He's so secretive." Such straightforward statements—
what we call linear explanations—communicate to the therapist, "Fix
him and our problems as a couple will be solved."

The therapist's task is to begin to formulate hypotheses as he joins
with the couple. As the therapist listens to the men discuss their problems and their origins, he is beginning to identify what mutual behaviors maintain them. The therapist remains in control of these early sessions by directing questions to each partner. For a couple to open up
raw emotions too quickly can be countertherapeutic and create an unsafe atmosphere. The task during this early stage of treatment is for the
couple to know that each partner will have an opportunity to express
his concerns. By remaining close to the couple and central during this
phase, the therapist can structure the session to help ensure that each
person is adequately heard.

Spontaneous interactions between the partners will often occur
during this stage of treatment, and experienced therapists can use these
enactments to create frames (i.e., images or insights) of how the couple

have constructed their relationship that maintains this homeostasis. For instance, in a relationship where the couple dynamic is underfunctioning–overfunctioning complementary behaviors, if one partner continues to complete the sentences of the other, the therapist might wonder aloud whether that behavior might account in part for the silent partner's underfunctioning. The experienced therapist might say, "I notice that, whenever I ask you a question, your partner answers. Let's hear from *him*. Perhaps that's why you spend so much time at the office. Do you ever feel unemployed at home?" The couple is already being educated to one of the basic tenets of structural family therapy, namely, that complementary behaviors create predictable patterns of interactions with predictable outcomes. However, for a therapist new to family therapy, we suggest that she make a mental note of the dynamic or even reflect her observation of the behavior to the couple and continue to focus on the history of the presenting problem. "When did you first notice his lack of interest in you?" or "Your partner says you work all the time. Is that how you view it?" are questions that will help to focus the session.

All couples struggle to create a relationship that meets the needs of each of the partners and identifies them as an entity separate from other systems. The reconfiguration of roles to accommodate each other's needs and the boundary making required to create a new family identity are challenging and stressful to both partners. What may be a surprise for a family therapist new to working with gay couples are both the similarities and differences of the presenting problems. Because there are few laws and so few institutionalized rituals that acknowledge and affirm the union between same-sex couples, gay couples have to make up the rules as they go along. Furthermore, most male couples have few role models to use when constructing their relationship. Gay men will often reject heterosexual couple norms for reasons related to politics because they believe those norms aren't relevant to their relationships. For instance, it is not uncommon for a gay couple to present in treatment with a disagreement over whether they should have a monogamous or an open relationship. Or a couple may be struggling with how to create complementary roles as a family, a presenting problem common to all couples but exacerbated for gay couples due to their isolation and lack of common norms.

The task of boundary making is a challenge for gay couples because frequently families of origin do not recognize the men as being a couple even when each of them is out to their families. Not being recognized as a couple creates split loyalties, as each man is often automatically drawn to remain loyal to his biological family. It is not uncommon for a therapist to discover that, even in a long-established gay couple, each man continues to separate and return to his family of origin for important holidays. This dynamic is destabilizing for a couple as they struggle to create a family identity with their own traditions and rituals. Just as a therapist would be surprised to discover this dynamic with a heterosexual couple, she should be curious as she questions the effect of the behavior on the integrity of a gay couple. If the clients have partnered siblings, the therapist might ask, "Do your siblings also leave their spouses during holidays?"

HISTORY OF THE RELATIONSHIP

Once each partner has identified why he has come to therapy, the therapist will want to take a history of the couple's relationship. Areas of interest for a systemic therapist include how did the couple meet; what attracted them to each other; what was their courtship like; do they have an anniversary date; have they had or do they plan to have a commitment ceremony; do they have an open or closed relationship; and do they have, or do they intend to adopt, children? If the therapist was working with a heterosexual couple, none of these questions (with the possible exception of that relating to monogamy) would appear novel. For a gay couple, the questions introduce therapeutic novelty as the therapist focuses on identifying the strengths of their relationship and simultaneously honors them as a couple. Furthermore, the therapist is gathering important information to make tentative hypotheses regarding what mutual behaviors maintain the couple's presenting problem. It is equally important for the therapist to know where a couple is developmentally in their life cycle. For instance, the tasks for a couple early in the stages of identity formation and boundary making differ markedly from those of a couple struggling to incorporate adolescents into a blended family.

Additionally and unique to working with same-sex couples, as the therapist takes the history of the gay couple's relationship, she begins to weave in questions that will provide her with information about each man's stage of gay identity development and his process of coming out. For example, if one or both of the men are closeted and not out to family or colleagues, a therapist will want to explore how that dynamic impacts them as a couple. Couples, straight and gay, benefit from community support, and isolation creates stress on the relationship. Clandestine relationships can initially be exciting because of their secretiveness, but eventually those relationships are at high risk due to their lack of supportive resources.

A CLINICAL EXAMPLE OF JOINING

A clinical example of an intake with a male couple will illustrate the initial joining phase. Don and Gerry have been in a relationship for the past 5 years. Don is a designer from a close-knit Italian Jewish family. Gerry is a successful realtor from an Irish Catholic family. Both men are in their early forties and recently began living together in Don's apartment. When the therapist asks why they have come to see him, they both complain about a lack of closeness in their relationship. When the therapist pushes each man to be more specific, Don says he is angry at what he describes as Gerry's dullness. Gerry (who initially called to make the appointment) then speaks at length about his concern over Don's recent abuse of the drug Ecstasy and his going to clubs on weekends with friends. Gerry is bewildered by Don's new behavior and fears for his health. Gerry also says he often feels excluded from Don's social life. What was apparent to the therapist as he joined with the couple was the parental quality of Gerry's complaints. Don initially said little— only that he was tired of leading a dull life with Gerry and that he intended to enjoy his life now that he was in his forties.

The therapist could take one of several paths at this stage. If he were to focus solely on the destabilizing and potentially deleterious effects of Don's drug usage and club attendance, he would have bought Gerry's explanation of the couple's problem: "Don's misbehaving." Making a mental note that Gerry's style appeared highly parental, the therapist chose to further explore the history of Don and Gerry's relationship. He wanted to know more about the men. How did they meet? The therapist knew he needed to gather more information about their dynamics as a couple if he was to understand what mutual behaviors had instigated and were maintaining Don's recent forays into the party circuit.

The men reported that they began dating when Gerry was in a heterosexual marriage. Initially their dating was secretive and consisted of romantic afternoon trysts and weekend dates. Eventually Gerry disclosed his bisexuality to his wife and revealed the affair that he and Don had been having for 2 years. Gerry said that his wife was not surprised with his revelation and had always suspected that he was bisexual. Gerry and his wife had married when they were both in college and had raised one son together, who was now a junior in high school. Gerry's main concern when he separated from his wife was how he could continue to be a father to his son. Gerry's wife agreed that they should separate so that they would both be free to pursue more fulfilling relationships. As the therapist continued to take Don and Gerry's history, he was thinking, "What is Don's new behavior intended to communicate to Gerry—and why *now*?"

Don continued to remain silent, and the therapist knew it was important to join with him. Using Don's words, the therapist said, "When did you begin to feel that Gerry was so dull?" Though still early in the first session, the therapist wanted to challenge the explicit message that Don was the problem to be fixed. The therapist began to challenge that frame by refocusing on Gerry's behavior. He expanded the problem to include how Gerry contributed to Don's going out on the party circuit.

Since moving in together 2 years ago, Don said that Gerry was emotionally less available and distracted with work. The therapist asked if Gerry's distancing was new behavior, and Don replied "No" but that, prior to his moving in, he had been very busy building his own career. Recently Don's reputation as a designer had become better established. Now that Gerry was living with him, Don was more aware of how distracted Gerry seemed. The therapist encouraged Don to tell Gerry specifically what bothered him. Don told Gerry that he was ready to break up the relationship. He was tired of feeling "like a mistress." When the therapist asked Gerry if he knew what Don meant, Gerry looked bewildered. He said that he thought Don was going through a mid-life crisis. Remaining central to control the session, the therapist asked Don if that was true. Don responded to Gerry, "If you're not going to be available, I'm going to enjoy my life and my friends. You can go back to your wife." The therapist said, "You mean his ex-wife?" Don said, "No, I mean his wife. They still vacation together. I'm the third wheel."

The probable meaning of Don's behavior had become clearer to the therapist as the nature of their problem unfolded. The therapist hypothesized that, though they had been together for several years, Don and

Gerry had never become a couple. While they had lived separately and while Don had been busy building his career, their parallel lives had not been a threat to Don. Now that they were living together and struggling to create an identity as a couple, they were doing the work of creating a home that they had previously postponed. Gerry, possibly reflecting his desire to parent his son, appeared to never have fully committed to a relationship with Don. Don, previously preoccupied in building his own career, was now ready to be closer to Gerry. The therapist also thought about where Gerry might be in his struggle to integrate his gay identity and what impact the disclosure of his sexual orientation might have had on his relationship with his son. The therapist chose to pursue a line of questioning that focused on the basic task of creating a couple identity.

LISTENING TO THE COUPLE'S SUBTEXT

In Chapter 3 we noted that the two tasks in becoming a couple are boundary making, or creating an identity, and accommodation. Though the couple's problem, as presented by Gerry, was Don's nightclubbing, the therapist's hypothesis was that this couple was struggling with issues common to blended families. The task for them was how to create a boundary and an identity separate from Gerry's former marriage. While Gerry needed to continue to communicate with his wife in order to parent his son, the task was for him to emotionally disconnect from her so that he was available to make a home with Don. Similarly, Don had needs for intimacy and affiliation in his relationship with Gerry that were not being met. The therapist wondered if Don's behavior was having the reverse effect of what he had actually wanted, that is, driving Gerry closer to his wife rather than pulling him into their partnership.

The therapist knew it was important to support Gerry's desire to parent his teenaged son and to maintain open channels of communication with his son's mother. He decided to highlight Gerry's strengths in his relationship with Don before he challenged him. "Don, you obviously fell in love with a very caring, responsible man who wants to be a good father to his son." Then he challenged Gerry's failure to disengage emotionally with his wife. "Gerry, is it possible, though, that Don is right? Do you still have one foot in your marriage with your wife? I wonder if you've unpacked your bags in your new home."

Gerry responded in a businesslike manner, "Oh, yes, I'm fully committed to being with Don." The therapist did not accept Gerry's reassurance. He continued with his inquiry as he wondered aloud why Don might be challenging Gerry. Gerry had difficulty understanding his partner's angst over his continued involvement with his wife.

At this point in the session the therapist, though aware that he was still in the joining phase with this couple and educating them to the interdependency of their behaviors, felt a pull to focus the session on Don's drug abuse. He was activated to intervene by the crisis that he feared could potentially destroy their relationship.[1] The therapist made a decision to intervene, aware that he felt pulled in two directions by Don's behavior. While wanting to support Don's voice and not take up the role of his parent, he knew that Don was using self-destructive tactics to capture his partner's attention. The therapist said, "I understand your wanting Gerry's attention, but why play Russian roulette to get it?" Don looked stunned. The therapist simply repeated his question. Don began by saying he had started going to circuit parties with some of his single friends because he was bored in his relationship with Gerry. At these all-night parties, hundreds of gay men gathered at a designated club in a highly sexualized environment. Drugs were everywhere at these parties, and Don regularly began to use Ecstasy, a drug that induced euphoria but more importantly, he said, gave him a feeling of "oneness" with his community.

The therapist hypothesized that Don was expressing his emotional loneliness by attending these parties—but, equally significant, he was endangering his health. His behavior was threatening to destabilize his relationship with Gerry as well. The therapist felt the need to challenge this destructive behavior. "Your drug usage can alter your brain's chemistry and result in long-term depression. You should find some less dangerous way to get Gerry's attention."

We take a firm position against the use of illicit drugs. Party drugs such as Ecstasy, Special K, and Crystal not only are self-destructive but also destabilize meaningful relationships. Although we believe the high

---

[1] This is a good example of when the therapist's theoretical knowledge could have interfered with his work as a clinician. Normally the structural therapist activates one partner to challenge the other instead of taking on the task himself. A therapist's decision to remain central and active in any given session may diminish the couple's ability to resolve their differences. Additionally, overly active therapists tend to burn out rapidly in clinical practice. As a rule, the therapist's red light should go on when he finds himself doing the work of the couple.

incidence of illicit drug abuse among a certain subset of gay men may be related to larger issues of loss from the AIDS epidemic and misconstrued self-medication in response to feelings of shame due to discrimination, the undeniable long-term deleterious effects of drug abuse may create a crisis for a family therapist. The drug abuse must be addressed immediately for treatment to be effective. In this case, the therapist had been "organized" by his expertise with substance abuse. He could not pursue his role as a structural family therapist and his usual stance of initially supporting a partner in challenging problematic behaviors of his significant other until he addressed Don's substance abuse.

Time was up and the session was over for that day. The therapist ended the session by summarizing his observations. The therapist said, "You're a couple struggling like many new couples to create a family. Gerry's love and commitment to his son is admirable, but I wonder if you have created a space for yourselves as a couple. Gerry, your wife has been the primary caretaker of your son, but you want to participate in your son's life. However, you appear to be struggling as to how you can do this and still stay connected with Don. Don, you had previously been focused on building your career and now want to change the rules of the relationship. Though focused on a desire to increase intimacy in your relationship, you seem to be caught in one dramatic, potentially self-destructive style of registering your loneliness. Rather than focusing on coming together as a couple, your behavior, Don, seems to have had the paradoxical effect of pushing Gerry further away."

The therapist then told the couple he thought they could benefit from couple treatment and he would work to help them find solutions to their problems. Both men agreed to come back. Before the session ended, the therapist made a verbal contract with the couple. The therapist said he would help Don to discover ways other than drug use for him to feel connected. Both men also agreed to set aside any talk of separation while in treatment. The therapist said that at the end of 12 sessions they would then pause and assess whether the treatment had been helpful. Both partners concurred.

Making a verbal contract with a couple new to treatment is a technique that we have found helpful with gay couples. When there are no civil or legal documents that bind a couple, separation can often be a knee-jerk response to conflict for men. For reasons stated earlier, we find that men often have an initial response to disconnect when confronted with conflict. Gay men are especially vulnerable to disengagement as a result of prior trauma. A therapist cannot work effectively if he feels that a couple may exercise the option to separate any time the treatment gets challenging. The threat of dissolution of a relationship effectively ties a therapist's hands. He cannot feel free to challenge a couple, knowing that a period of discomfort is normal in structural treatment as a couple struggles to discover new ways to relate. We use this contract most often with male couples, but it also can be effective when working with heterosexual couples who are tenuously connected.

A week later, Don and Gerry came into the therapist's office looking upset. The therapist asked how the couple were doing and if they had any thoughts about the prior session. Without a pause, Don blasted into Gerry, accusing him of still being married to his wife. Gerry's response was to become silent as his face turned red. Using this spontaneous interaction, the therapist reflected the dynamic that he had just observed. The therapist chose the image of a baseball bat. He asked Don if it was necessary to use a baseball bat to get Gerry's attention. The image that the therapist used was intended to convey a mixed message to Don. The therapist was supporting both Don's masculinity and his assertiveness as he simultaneously challenged his harshness. The therapist was conveying the message "Stand up for what you believe in, but can't you be more soft?"

The therapist asked if Don could speak to Gerry "without using a baseball bat." This time, Don was able to speak about his loneliness while using less confrontational language. He did not attack his partner as the therapist coached him to use language that revealed his vulnerability. Gerry was able to hear his partner's pain and appeared less threatened. However, Gerry still responded defensively and concretely by saying that the real estate market was down and that it was not a good time to sell the property that he and his wife jointly owned. The therapist told Don that he thought Gerry could hear him now and that he might want to continue to use more of this softer language. Don said jokingly, "If I don't hit him with a baseball bat, he won't hear me. He falls asleep instantly." Both men laughed at the imagery.

Although Don and Gerry were just beginning couple treatment, the therapist had used a spontaneous enactment to unbalance the couple. His challenge had helped the men to understand where they might be stuck in the relationship that they had constructed. Yet, the therapist still needed to learn more about them as a couple, to understand what their early courtship was like, what initially attracted them to each other, and what they enjoyed doing together as a couple. At this juncture the therapist wanted to convey to them that he had heard their problem, he would return to it, but he also needed to know more about them as a couple.

The therapist said, "I hear you struggling to become a family separate and unique from your former relationships. Don, you feel that Gerry's emotional loyalties are still with his wife and son. I think that you're expressing your anger by attending circuit parties. But that's only half the story. Gerry, you're alarmed and confused by Don's recent desire to go out on the singles party circuit and feel that your relationship is threatened. However, you haven't been able to convince him that, along with your son, he is your top priority." They nodded in agreement that the therapist had gotten it right.

Wanting to discover more of their strengths, the therapist continued: "We'll return to this, but first I would like to get to know you as a couple. Tell me how you met. Do you remember your first date?" They both smiled and nodded their heads in agreement. Each man told a story of seeing the other at a tennis club that they belonged to. Every day at the club, they would exchange glances. Gradually Gerry got up the courage to talk with Don, and they began to have lunch together. Lunch developed into a romantic and sexual relationship that continued for a couple of years.

Both men talked about coming from large families. Don said he was close to his family, and Gerry reported that he saw his family only occasionally. Don's family had accepted his homosexuality since late adolescence, and he had always introduced his dates or partners to his family. Gerry's family was not aware of his bisexuality, and he had few gay friends prior to meeting Don. As they began to date, they remained isolated, due both to the secretiveness of their relationship and the limited time they had with each other. The therapist also learned that, due to the irregularity of their dating, from the beginning both men agreed that they would have an open relationship. Gerry was still with his wife, and Don spent most of the week by himself.

After Gerry came out to his wife, the couple agreed to an amicable separation and Gerry was free to openly live with Don. What previously was a clandestine relationship, electrified by the secretiveness of their meetings, now became more mundane. Additionally, although Gerry was now free to move in with Don, it appeared to the therapist that his primary emotional ties remained with his former wife and son. The men's social life revolved around Gerry's wife and son. Both concurred that the 16-year-old son, who visited them regularly at their apartment, had been surprisingly accepting of their relationship. However, the two men had yet to develop interests of their own, and they lacked a supportive community of mutual friends.

Furthermore, although Don loved to travel, he had largely discontinued optional travel since meeting Gerry. Gerry, busy raising a family and building a career, had few recreational interests. As a couple they had not found a common bond other than their physical attraction to each other. The honeymoon was over, and the work of building a long-term relationship had just begun.

This first example of joining helps to exemplify the nonlinear nature of structural family therapy. Although we describe the model in terms of three distinct phases (joining, enactments, and unbalancing), rarely do cases unfold so neatly. As this case demonstrates, enactments may erupt spontaneously as the therapist takes the history. The therapist instantly became inducted into the system and momentarily was activated to become a savior. The model is important to keep in mind, though, as it helps a therapist organize a map to maneuver through the maze of issues that families and couples present with.

After two sessions, we could now draw a structural map that reflects the therapist's hypotheses about the couple's system and that he could use to help guide him in his work with the couple (see Figure 4.2). Gerry's primary affiliation appears to be with his wife and son. Don turns to outside activities to occupy himself in Gerry's absence in

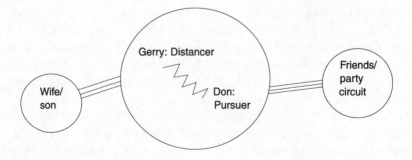

FIGURE 4.2. Map of Don and Gerry's mutual problem and complementary roles. Parallel lines represent overinvolvement of the men with nonpartners, and the jagged line indicates conflict between the two men.

lieu of confronting Gerry with his loneliness. Gerry, not feeling that he has a home with Don, stays close to his ex-wife. The problem can be reframed as not a linear one of Don's acting out but one that is maintained by the couple's complementary behaviors. Gerry maintains his emotional ties to his wife to obtain an intimacy that he has not yet gotten from Don. Don goes to friends and clubs to avoid confrontation and to get his affiliative needs met. The map reflects the complexity of their dynamics and suggests possible interventions that could challenge the couple's status quo. If Gerry were to dissolve his marital ties with his wife entirely, he would be more available to Don. If Don could speak to his partner in a less combative manner, Gerry might move closer to him. And, if Don were not going outside the relationship to fulfill his needs for affiliation and moved closer to Gerry, he would be less lonely and resentful.

Their behavior illustrates the nature of circular causality. Notice that the therapist did not choose to enter the couple's system by challenging their open relationship policy. The couple had agreed to this arrangement since the early days of their relationship, and both men appeared to be comfortable with the agreement. Neither was it necessary for the therapist to enter into the realm of Gerry's possible foreclosure of his gay identity development. Nor did it appear necessary to include Gerry's son or wife in the treatment, as both men were in agreement about the father's continued involvement with his son and the son appeared accepting of the men's relationship.

THE CARETAKER AND HIS PATIENT

Another couple will further help illustrate the joining process. This couple's presenting problem was that one of the men wanted to open up the relationship to multiple sexual partners, while his partner refused to engage in any conversation about the possibility of being nonmonogamous. The couple consisted of Ernie and James, two men in their late 20s who had been together for 2 years. They arrived for their first session on bicycles, each of them wearing distinctly different outfits. Ernie was in athletic biking clothes and James wore loose-fitting attire. Both men were out of breath from peddling from the Williamsburg section of Brooklyn. They stumbled into the therapist's office and plopped themselves down on the sofa.

Before the therapist had an opportunity to ask even a single question, Ernie disclosed the impasse that had been reached over whether they should open up their relationship to multiple sexual partners. Ernie said that he wanted a nonmonogamous relationship and that James refused to even discuss the possibility.

If taken at face value, the dilemma for them as a couple seemed to be a simple one, though one having profound implications for the relationship. The problem was that James unilaterally opposed Ernie's idea and refused to engage in any discussion of the topic. As Ernie had scheduled the session and led the argument to open their relationship, the implicit message to the therapist was clear: "Help me change James's mind and all will be well in our relationship."

During this early stage of treatment the therapist wanted to convey to Ernie and James that he had heard their problem as he continued to speculate how the issue of monogamy might be symptomatic of some larger systemic issue in the couple's relationship. This is a very delicate stage of treatment. The couple and therapist are just getting to know one another and to build an alliance through the joining process. James and Ernie had come for treatment because they had a concrete problem that they wanted the therapist to resolve for them. The therapist needed to communicate to Ernie and James that, while he respected their dilemma, he still needed to remain open to discovering what the inability to resolve this conflict meant for them as a couple.

The structural family therapist saw their problem as a possible metaphor for how they made decisions throughout their relationship. He speculated to himself that he could enter their relationship at any of many junctures and he would most likely discover a similar dynamic at work. If he got caught up in concrete problem-solving tasks, he would risk the danger of being inducted into their system. And if he became part of their system, his hands would be tied to effectively challenge their currently limited way of relating to each other. The temptation might also exist for the therapist to get caught up in a discussion of the political ideology of an open versus a closed relationship. While remaining mindful of all these possibilities, the therapist needed to discover the meaning of the presenting problem for this couple.

The task for the structural therapist at this early stage of joining is not only to identify the area of conflict but also to explore it as a symptom of what mutual behaviors maintain and preclude a resolution. The therapist simply said, "I hear you're stuck negotiating an issue that many gay couples struggle with. Tell me, how long have you had this conflict?" After ascertaining that this was a relatively new problem in their relationship, the therapist then questioned the couple to find out if either man was currently involved with someone else. There are several ways that a therapist could gather this information. Some family therapists meet with each person alone to ascertain if there is any information such as an extramarital affair that the therapist should know about. We advise against using this strategy during the early stages of treatment, as the therapist is then caught in the dilemma of what to do with this secret. (Cases of domestic violence can be the exception to this policy not to meet separately with the partners during this phase, as the therapist may need to create a safe place for the abused person to disclose the violence.)

In this case both men denied any extramarital affairs. The therapist then said that he would return to this important issue but he first wanted to know more about them as a couple. Here again, the therapist is gathering more information to ascertain the complementary roles that preclude resolution of their presenting problem and maintain homeostasis in the system. In some ways Ernie and James's problem can be seen as learning to listen and to accommodate each other's needs. They could have just as easily have been caught, as Trudy and Jed were, in a disagreement about whether they should live in the suburbs or the city.

The therapist proceeded to take a history of Ernie and James's relationship. Most couples like to tell the story of their relationship. It often brings them back to an earlier time in their relationship when they were happy. Often, as the honeymoon period ends, a couple experiences conflict as they struggle to learn to accommodate each other's needs. They experience stress as they acknowledge their differences and learn to become a "we," in which individual differences are considered secondary to the well-being of the relationship. Male couples often interpret this stressful transition as symptomatic of unresolvable differences that demonstrate that they are not meant to be a couple. Male couples often break up during these inevitable transitional periods. The task for the couple is to learn how to mediate their differences. It can be a reality test when two men newly in love realize they need to be able to tolerate that their needs are not identical. For gay men who lack dating experience, this realization can prove to be a particularly threatening experience. The therapist needs to normalize the process as he helps a couple to discover their strengths to maneuver through this new phase of their relationship.

In exploring how Ernie and James courted each other and ascertaining how quickly they became a committed couple, the therapist hoped he would get an idea of how solid a foundation they had to build their relationship on. Couples who have experienced a period of bliss during the early stages of their relationship have memories that can give them strength and hope. If they are able to resolve their differences, they may be able to recapture the early loving experiences. Conversely, couples that committed to each other *without* any period of courtship may have to go back in their life cycle together to build a stronger foundation for a long-term relationship.

The therapist realized that Ernie and James' complementary traits had been suggested in their behavior during the first few minutes of the session. Ernie was the smaller of the two men, gregarious and emotionally expressive. Casually dressed in form-fitting biking clothes, he was quite handsome. His partner, James, much taller than Ernie, sat in the therapist's office in baggy draw-string pants and a fisherman's tunic, one leg underneath him in a half-lotus position. He was poised as he revealed that he was a yoga practitioner and vegetarian.

While Ernie expressed his intense desire to open the relationship, James remained quiet and serene throughout this part of the session. His tranquil facial expression suggested sympathy for Ernie's plight, but it was clear James was unwilling to consider that Ernie's desire for an open relationship might somehow be related to larger issues in their relationship. Ernie appeared to be most perturbed by James's unwillingness to even engage in dialogue on the subject.

The therapist took a history of their courtship. Ernie and James told the therapist how they had met on a blind date. Both reported being immediately attracted to the other. Ernie next told of a significant event that happened in their lives 6 months after they started dating. Ernie was in a life-threatening bicycle accident, and James immediately took up the role of Ernie's caretaker. Ernie was grateful for James's ability to nurse him back to good health. Ernie spoke tearfully of the vulnerability and love that he had experienced for James, being cared for by another man for the first time in his adult life. Both men agreed that the time when Ernie was recovering from his injuries was when they had felt the happiest. James had moved into Ernie's apartment during that period, and each man felt as though he had found a soul mate in the other. Despite periods of pain for Ernie, both described this period as idyllic. For the first time, the therapist experienced their tenderness for each other, and he thought that this might be a good omen for the couple's ability to survive their current crisis.

When the therapist asked what each man did for a living, James became the spokesman for the couple as he responded that they were going through a difficult financial period. James was a designer who supplemented his income by tending bar a couple of nights a week. Ernie said that he was currently on disability. Prior to his bicycle accident, he had trained as a drummer and had just started playing in local clubs. He had supplemented his earnings as a musician by waiting on tables. Since his accident, however, Ernie had not gone back to either playing the drums or waiting on tables. The therapist asked Ernie how his disability contributed to their financial difficulties. James responded for Ernie and reassured the therapist that they were coping. Despite a large credit card debt, James did not expect Ernie to work. Ernie seemed less worried than James about finances. He reported that his family contributed to his support.

As Ernie was approaching his thirtieth birthday and appeared in good health, the therapist wondered about his financial dependence upon his biological family. The therapist asked Ernie whether he was currently unable to work or whether had he been advised by his doctor to stay off his feet. Ernie said that he was free to physically do anything at this point but that inertia had set in and he felt depressed. When the therapist asked for more details, Ernie reported feeling depressed for the past few months. The therapist then commented, "Depression is often anger that gets turned in on the self. Who are you angry at?" Both men stared at the therapist as if he had just sprouted another head. When the therapist repeated his question, Ernie was at a loss for an answer and just laughed. The therapist looked inquiringly at James, who simply shrugged his shoulders. "Ernie," the therapist said, "maybe your desire to open up the relationship is an attempt to communicate something to James?"

The therapist was moving quickly for this early stage of treatment. We often work at several levels simultaneously. A couple gains insight in how they have co-constructed their relationship as they begin to experiment with new behaviors. The therapist's role is to introduce to a couple the reality that their behavior does not exist in isolation but is organized in many ways. At this moment, the therapist was focusing on Ernie and James's dyadic system and the mutual behaviors that might explain their crisis. The therapist chose not to enter into their experience with larger systems for now, to explore how the couple's behavior might be affected by these systems—their families, the presence or absence of social support systems, and their experiences with the majority culture. The initial role for a structural family therapist is to identify the complementary behaviors observed in the session and to unbalance the partners' dance by encouraging the couple to begin experimenting with new ways of relating. It is neither necessary nor even desirable for the therapist to explore each individual's experience of the world. During this early stage of treatment both the therapist and the couple might be overwhelmed by such details.

Although only 30 minutes into the session, the therapist was beginning to have sufficient information to draw a map of how this couple might have constructed their relationship. They had met and fallen in love quickly, not an unusual phenomenon for many couples, irrespective of sexual orientation. But the process of courtship for gay couples is often attenuated, at best. Without social rituals and civil ceremonies common to heterosexual couples, gay couples are freer to both form and dissolve relationships spontaneously. Often gay men find themselves in intimate relationships without having gone through the process of courting, wherein couples often create a culture of how to negotiate decision making. These common experiences in heterosexual dating rituals help a couple to build the confidence that they have the resources to endure moments of conflict in their relationship.

James and Ernie had been catapulted into their relationship by an unusual emergency that had occurred early in the life cycle of their relationship—Ernie's life was threatened and James responded by becoming his caretaker. James told the therapist how, as a practitioner of meditation and yoga, he had taught Ernie to use these practices to speed his recovery. The therapist thought to himself that, in the process of being cared for, Ernie had become James's patient. This is not an uncommon complementary construction for a couple and one that worked—that is, so long as Ernie still needed a caretaker. The therapist hypothesized that the relationship had become rigidified around this limited definition of who these men were to each other. James was overfunctioning in the relationship and Ernie was underfunctioning. James's caretaker and teacher roles appeared to give him an elevated position in their relationship, while Ernie's dependent role kept him in a one-down status.

Extreme differences between partners are not uncommon in gay relationships and can often be sources of strength and richness for a couple. Older–younger, wealthy–poor, mixed ethnicity or race, and teacher–student are just some of the possible complementary roles. Couples thrive on differences and yet simultaneously they need to have sufficient flexibility and a shared set of values that overlap and allow them to develop a common language. The therapist drew an initial map (Figure 4.3) for himself where he thought James and Ernie were stuck and could create a possible reframe of their problem.

Some family therapists might undertake to request of the partners a *genogram* (McGoldrick & Gerson, 1985) at this stage of the treatment to ascertain how James's and Ernie's families of origin prepared them for these roles of caretaker and patient. Among other things, genograms provide a therapist with valuable information that is helpful in ascertaining and assessing each partner's values. Usually one partner listens and takes in the information while the other talks about his family of origin. This task maintains a therapist's centrality in the session and generally minimizes affect.

In contrast, the structural family therapist intervenes more directly and helps the couple unbalance the behavior enacted in the therapeutic session. Ernie and James's therapist wanted to maintain intensity at this juncture in treatment, and he continued to focus on the system that the couple had mutually constructed. He was organized by his belief that getting "unstuck" and expanding their currently limited roles would potentially have a trickle-down healing effect in their individual lives. The therapist decided he would not explore each partner's individual

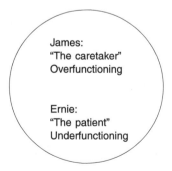

James:
"The caretaker"
Overfunctioning

Ernie:
"The patient"
Underfunctioning

FIGURE 4.3. Structural map with rigid boundaries and the absence of a social support network.

history until the middle stage of treatment and only then if he was unable to unbalance the "here and now" dynamics of the interactions he was observing.

The therapist created a frame that tested his hypothesis that James and Ernie were caught in caretaker–patient complementary roles by the language that he used. "You have constructed a very special relationship of a loving caretaker and a grateful patient. Do you ever want to break out of the role of patient, Ernie? Is it difficult to have sex with your guru?"

Both men looked startled at first. While James looked totally confused, Ernie slowly nodded his head in agreement and said, "Yes! He always talks to me like I'm 12 years old! " As the session was about to end, the therapist made a mental note of James's confusion over his challenge. The therapist had created an initial frame that expanded Ernie and James's linear problem. He still needed to join with them further, knowing he would return to this limited definition they had constructed of each other in the next session. He wanted to gather more information about them as a couple, but the time was up for the first session. He asked the couple if they had any questions about this first session.

Ernie wondered if the therapist was opposed to open relationships. The therapist said he had worked with couples who have successfully negotiated an open relationship but they had first come up with a specific set of rules governing sexual encounters. The negotiations required each partner to listen to the other and be willing to accommodate himself to the other's needs for safety and security. He also said that many gay couples intellectually approve of the concept but have difficulty in implementing the rules. He added: "Sometimes, opening a relationship can be an avoidance of conflict in the relationship related to feelings of 'deadness' between the partners."

Ernie and James seemed to be mulling over this information as the therapist said he would like to schedule another session before they made a therapeutic contract. We often take two sessions to make an assessment of a couple, particularly if we are limited to a one-hour intake. In this case, the therapist wasn't sure that Ernie and James were willing to give up their limiting but well-established roles. James seemed to be committed to his hierarchical role as "keeper of the truth," and Ernie's lifelong financial dependence on his family, and now James, did not bode well for freeing himself from his subordinate position as patient.

Complementary roles and worry over the rigidity of these roles are common phenomena among couples in Western culture. However, roles also create order and efficiency in systems. Complementary roles become problematic when one or both partners feel limited and the system is insufficiently flexible to allow for new growth. Recently many heterosexual relationships have undergone a redefinition of roles as women increasingly experience more equitable earning power. The high divorce rate in the United States reflects, among other things, stresses related to renegotiated roles in family systems. However, for male couples there are no traditional role models to emulate as a starting point. They are creating and negotiating their roles as they construct their relationships.

Historically, some gay couples in an effort to avoid conflict mimicked traditional heterosexual role models, one partner taking up the "male" tasks and the other assuming the "woman's" role. This generally is as disastrous for long-term gay couples as it is for heterosexual ones. Few of us want to exclusively define ourselves as homemaker, laundry doer, or housecleaner. Sometimes we want to be the driver and at other times the passenger. Healthy relationships often have this flexibility.

SECOND SESSION: JOINING CONTINUES

During the next session the therapist chose not to return immediately to the rigid roles James and Ernie had constructed. Instead, he began to focus on what kind of support systems the couple had. Finding out what type of a support system a couple has, who honors them as a couple, is extremely important for any new couple but critical for the well-being of gay couples. Many gay men are not out to their biological families or, if out, may have been ostracized from participating in family activities. It's important for a therapist to ascertain who supports them as a couple. Do they have either gay-affirmative straight allies or other gay couples they socialize with and who can normalize the difficult transition from being single to becoming a "we"?

In Ernie and James's second session, they reported having only a few gay and straight friends, but they had no other couples in their support network. Moreover, their primary social relationships were with friends each of them had prior to becoming a couple. Essentially, they were trying to negotiate this new territory on their own. Therapy, as is often true for gay couples, could potentially be a healing experience that both mediated their differences and supported their togetherness. The treatment becomes a safe haven as the couple explores ways to obtain more social support.

James was estranged from his family. He had come out to his conservative Christian mother when he was in college, and her response was, "Don't tell your grandmother; it would kill her." She refused to talk about his sexual orientation and discouraged him from bringing any of his gay friends home. His father was deceased, and his only sibling, a sister, left home after high school and lived on the West Coast. Although he was not estranged from her, they had little contact, as her husband didn't like "fags."

Ernie, in turn, presented a totally different family story. He had been out to his parents and siblings since high school. They knew James and accepted him into their home as Ernie's friend. Ernie brought James home for major holidays, and the men shared the same bedroom. Perhaps an indication of a lack of acceptance of Ernie's sexual orientation, both men laughed as they reported that Ernie's mother was so comfortable with their friendship that she didn't even bother to knock on their bedroom door before coming in to see what they wanted for breakfast.

The therapist began to get a feeling of a large, warm, loving family—but one with no boundaries. "Do they recognize you as a couple?" the therapist asked Ernie. "Maybe they just think of you as friends. Why otherwise would she walk unannounced into your bedroom? Unless she's voyeuristic . . . is she a voyeur?" Both men laughed at the absurdity of the therapist's questions but seemed perplexed. The therapist then asked, "How does she refer to you as a couple?" Ernie responded, "She doesn't refer to us." James added, "She simply calls us 'the boys'." The therapist remarked that he thought that was strange, and he wondered if she referred to Ernie's sister and brother-in-law as children too.

With this additional information, the therapist confirmed his hypothesis that this couple was struggling both to expand the relationship and accommodate each other's needs and to create an identity as a couple—two of the primary tasks during the early stages of creating a family. He wondered aloud about the meaning of Ernie's parents never accepting the fact that he was in the process of creating his own family. The transition from biological family of origin to adult family of choice can be problematic for many couples. The lack of any ritual to honor

Ernie and James's relationship and the isolation that they were experiencing was destabilizing the couple. The therapist wondered if Ernie's family's desexualizing his relationship with James was homophobia or a desire to maintain Ernie's status as their son.

As the therapist continued taking a history of this couple's relationship, he then returned to the topic of how they were managing to cope with their financial difficulties. Finances are a hot topic for most couples. Prenuptial agreements represent one way that couples express their fears around commitment and dependency. Male couples are often reticent to merge their resources. The obvious reason is the lack of legal protection due to the absence of laws providing protection for same-sex couples. However, the merging of one's financial resources with another person's also represents a permanent commitment to the relationship and an explicit dependency on each other.

Ernie and James were struggling to create an identity and to devise an equitable division of labor in their relationship. Not surprisingly, it turned out that the inequitable arrangement of their finances closely mirrored their struggles as a couple. James reiterated that they were having financial difficulties since Ernie's accident and had accumulated several thousand dollars in credit card debt. Ernie continued to appear less concerned about the status of their finances. When the therapist asked how they dealt with expenses, Ernie said that they each had separate checking accounts and contributed monthly to a common household account. The therapist asked again how their financial difficulties had been exacerbated by Ernie's accident. James repeated that he was the sole wage earner in the family, working two jobs.

Ernie gave a different response to the therapist's question, "I don't worry. My parents give me money." The therapist was surprised and questioned him further. He asked if they were wealthy or if they had given him a trust fund? He said, "No, they're middle-class, but they've supported me ever since I had the accident." The therapist was curious about this arrangement, as Ernie appeared healthy and reported that, other than feeling occasional fatigue, he had recovered from his accident. James added an interesting anecdote. Prior to his accident, Ernie's father had told James that he felt his son should be subsidized. He didn't want Ernie to work too hard, as he was struggling to be an artist.

The therapist felt caught here. He didn't wish to impose his own work ethics unduly on the couple, and yet he felt that Ernie was being held hostage by a conflictual message. Ernie, though depressed, was physically healthy. He resented the infantalized role he had with James and perhaps with his parents. Both James and Ernie's father were telling Ernie not to be self-supporting. We believe Freud was right when he noted that work is one way that we build our self-esteem. Given this contradiction, the therapist decided to explore the issue further. Ernie readily agreed that, ever since he had left home, his family had insisted on contributing to his support. " They think that, as an artist, I shouldn't have to worry constantly about money."

The therapist thought that Ernie's relationship to his family was roughly identical to the dependent but complementary relationship that he and James had constructed. The therapist began to wonder if his family's money might not be a financial umbilical cord that kept Ernie tied to his family. This umbilical cord might partially explain the difficulty that the couple was having in creating their own identity.

The issue of finances differs from one family culture to another. Some families are very generous and believe that young couples shouldn't have to struggle as they establish a new household. Financial support can be given to ease the hardship for a young couple. However, as a systems therapist, one always wonders whether there aren't strings attached to the financial aid. Does a new couple intend to remain loyal to the clan providing the financial aid? With Ernie and James, the therapist had a hunch that the contract that Ernie had implicitly made with his family was to never leave home. If the parents had lived closer to New York or were conveniently able to visit, the therapist might have encouraged Ernie to invite them in for a session to explore this possibility.

As the hour was nearly up for the second session, the therapist wanted to leave time to discuss a treatment contract. He summarized the issues and attempted to describe the struggle that Ernie and James appeared to be having in creating an identity. "All couples struggle—as the two of you are doing—to create an identity that says you are a unit distinct from other families. In the very early stages of becoming a couple, you appeared to have created roles in response to Ernie's health crisis. Those roles of caretaker and patient served you then, but they may be too restrictive now. You both appear motivated to discover new ways of relating to each other. Ernie, your wish to open the relationship to multiple sexual partners after being together for 2 years comes at an interesting time in your relationship. As I said at the end of our last session, some couples negotiate that kind of an agreement and report not feeling anxious. It doesn't appear that you're ready for that kind of a relationship." James interrupted and said he might be willing to discuss the possibilities, or at least listen to Ernie's point of view.

The therapist reinforced James' newfound flexibility. "I think it's important that Ernie knows you're willing to listen to him. But I would like to ask the two of you to shelve the monogamy issue for now. I think that you could benefit from couple treatment, and I think that we could work well together. Let's meet for a few sessions and see what meaning the monogamy issue has for the relationship. It seems too soon for us to know whether opening your relationship will destabilize it. I'd like to see you at this same time next week. Is that agreeable? Do you have any questions?" Neither Ernie nor James had questions, and they agreed to enter treatment, seemingly relieved by the therapist's summarization and support.

REVIEW OF THE JOINING PHASE OF TREATMENT

The therapist had met with each of the two couples for two sessions, and he now had some specific hypotheses that he would begin to test for each couple during the next stage of treatment. During the initial sessions, as he joined with each couple, he wanted to get a sense of who they were and what kind of a relationship they had established. As he joined with each couple and took their history, he began to create images, or mental maps, that expanded their presenting problem from a fairly simplistic (i.e., linear) one to one that was maintained primarily through *mutual* interaction. As the therapist began to educate each couple to the systemic concept that no problem exists in isolation, he simultaneously created an atmosphere of trust.

Tensions inevitably surfaced during the sessions as each couple came to confront their areas of conflict. The therapist did not discourage this tension; if sessions become too pleasant and too comfortable, a couple will experience insufficient anxiety to be motivated to risk experimentation with new behaviors, and the status quo will be maintained. If the couple doesn't drop out of treatment, the sessions will become flat and the therapist will begin to experience boredom, as might also the partners.

As the therapist took Ernie and James's history, it became clear that the couple had gotten stuck in their development by allowing the roles they had constructed when Ernie had his life-threatening accident to become too rigid. Both men were possibly predisposed to those roles from earlier experiences in their families. Structural family therapy is especially healing for marginalized populations such as gay couples because of its focus on the activation of dormant (i.e., latent) resources (Minuchin & Nichols, 1993). Rather than focusing on pathology or a dysfunctional past, we initially focus on activating strengths within the system. Ernie was currently underfunctioning in his relationship with his partner, but he has the capacity to be more resourceful if the context that organizes his behavior demands it. James's overfunctioning minimizes the contributions that Ernie needs to make to their relationship. If James were to become less active, Ernie would have to take up the complementary role of becoming more active. For a structural family therapist, the task of treatment is now to create a supportive environ conducive to change in the "here and now" reality of the session. During the next stage of treatment, enactments are an opportunity for the therapist and the couple to experience the complementary roles that they have constructed.

Avoidance of conflict is a common dynamic for most male couples. Disagreement arouses the primitive instinct of "fight or flight," and gay male couples often disengage rather than risk conflict. The therapist's expansion of Ernie and James's problem to make it an interpersonal dynamic created tension, but the therapist encouraged the men to stay connected as they began to negotiate a resolution. Perhaps if Ernie could challenge James constructively, he would become less depressed and more powerful in the relationship. But his decision unilaterally to broach the subject of opening the relationship so that he could experience more equality promised potentially to threaten their relationship. Both men were not addressing core issues in their relationship, specifically, the rigidity of the roles that they had constructed and the absence of a distinct identity for the two as a couple. Additionally, they would need to construct a social support system that honored their commitment to each other.

In the case of Don and Gerry, by the second session the therapist had also created a mental map of their relationship that he could explore with the couple. Although the issue as presented by Gerry was Don's recent interest in illicit drugs and the party circuit, once again the therapist reinterpreted the symptom to include its relational aspects. Thus, Don's behavior was in response to Gerry's lack of attention to

him. Gerry was in many ways still married to his former wife. Don's acting out had not been effective if he wanted to pull Gerry closer to him.
In fact, it was having the reverse effect. The work for the therapist
would be to create a safe environment in treatment that would first
magnify this dynamic and to then encourage the men to challenge it.
The therapist needed to create an atmosphere conducive for Don to tell
Gerry about his loneliness for him. The "baseball bat" was a metaphor
created by the therapist as he introduced language to magnify and unbalance this dynamic. Don's bat that he was taking to the relationship to
get his partner's attention was destructive. Essential to doing structural
therapy is the therapist's belief that the couple have both the desire and
the potential resources for a more satisfying relationship. How to create
and maintain a therapeutic atmosphere that is conducive to change as
the partners experiment with novelty is the focus of the next chapter.

CHAPTER FIVE

Enactments

Identifying Complementary Roles

In the preceding chapter we focused on the essential tasks during joining of history taking and structural mapping as a family therapist begins to reformulate a couple's presenting problem. Joining to create a therapeutic alliance with clients is common to all forms of therapy, and most therapists are adept at this. Once a therapist has taken a history and has a tentative map of a couple's style of relating, it is time to make the transition to the enactment stage of treatment to confirm her hypotheses.

A couple generally comes to family treatment with an individual linear understanding of the issues that are causing them stress, "the presenting problem." Enactments (Minuchin, 1981; Nichols, 1997; Nichols & Fellenberg, 2000) create opportunities for a therapist to observe the limited way a couple interact and help a couple expand their understanding of their problem, leading them to new, more satisfying, interactions. The structural therapist's task is to help the couple gain insight into what mutual behaviors prevent them from resolving their dilemma. In creating an enactment to observe how a couple relate, a therapist initiates, directs, and ends the interaction so that she is able to reframe their presenting problem to include the interpersonal dynamics that serve to maintain it.

Although the therapist generally initiates the enactments, they can occur spontaneously. They provide the therapist with a partial *in vivo* experience of how a couple has constructed their relationship. The word "partial" is used because the behavior that the therapist observes is a limited view of the couple's reality. Staged enactments are specific to structural family therapy and are often the most challenging phase of treatment for a new family therapist. When staging an enactment, the therapist goes from a proximal interactive role with a couple to a more distant intermediate position in order to observe their dynamics. Even for experienced family therapists, the fear arises that, since the enactment increases affect in the session, the therapist might lose control of the session. But it is precisely this affect and the interpersonal behaviors occurring during the enactments that the therapist needs most to observe.

As the therapist plans for a couple to interact, the therapist should first position the couple so they can face each other. If the couple are seated on a sofa, the therapist should ask one of the partners to move so that they can look at each other as they talk. In moving a couple so they face each other, the therapist is taking an intermediate position that discourages either partner from engaging her as she encourages them to interact with each other.

Next, the therapist asks a couple to talk about a specific issue with each other. Most couples will focus on a global problem in their relationship that may or may not relate to their presenting problem. The therapist will need to help the couple define the specific problem so that they can focus on a particular aspect of their relationship. The purpose of the enactment is for the therapist to experience the limited way the partners have defined and constructed interactions with each other. The therapist is then able to reflect back to the couple the interaction that she has just observed. The therapist is not so much critiquing the content of what the couple says as she is assessing a couple's style of relating to each other—their tone and affect, and their implicit assumptions about each other.

The philosophy that informs this phase of treatment is that people are more complex and resourceful than their initial presentation of themselves. Couples often become stuck in a predictable dance that they do together repeatedly. As an example, the man who initially appeared as the answer to a partner's dreams, due to the his self-sufficiency and independence, may end up getting labeled as the "cold withholding one" when the honeymoon stage of the relationship is over. What was once an asset early in the couple's relationship can become a liability. As the lonely partner becomes dissatisfied, he will attempt to change their relational style. If his independent partner is flexible, the couple can expand their repertoire of behaviors so that the lonely partner feels more connected. If the system is rigid, however, the couple will experience stress and conflict. It is at this stage of their relationship that the couple will often seek treatment.

Structural family therapy is a health-driven intervention. The structural therapist is observing the system to identify where the couple is caught in their complementary roles and to expand their way of relating in the belief that the couple has greater, if dormant, resources available if called upon. For instance, if the therapist is working with a couple where one partner complains that the other has an inability to experience closeness, one of the first questions that a therapist might ask is "What are the exceptions to the rule?" The therapist's thinking that informs the question is the belief that a couple's inability to express intimacy needs is a limited definition of who they are within a specific context; there may be other contexts where intimacy needs can be safely expressed. During enactments, the task for the therapist is to identify which circular behaviors serve to maintain the couple's presenting problem, and the couple's choice of context and topic are all-important in setting up the enactment.

Let's track a session to illustrate enactments that a therapist did with Luke and Fred, a couple who were in their mid-30s. The problem they presented to the therapist was that they could never resolve differences, and their arguments were frequently escalating to the point where Fred would threaten to break up the relationship. Fred's position was that Luke made him so anxious and angry when he disagreed with him that he became physically ill, resulting in his inability to concentrate at work. When the therapist asked Luke if he knew what he did that made his partner so anxious, he said that Fred's problem was that he was "too controlling." Both men were highly agitated, each blaming the other for their problems. This generalized complaint is not uncommon, but the therapist needed to gather more specific information to more fully understand the genesis of this couple's distress.

As the therapist took a history of their relationship, he discovered they had met when the younger of the two men, Luke, had been doing his social work training in a hospital where his future partner, Fred, was a staff physician. When the therapist asked what they had initially found attractive in each other, Fred volunteered how enamored he was of Luke's looks, intelligence, and curiosity. Luke described Fred as being strong, bold, attractive, and a "fountain of knowledge." Their descriptions of each other suggest an elegant example of the complementary roles of teacher–student, a dynamic that often works well until the student wants to graduate and think on his own.

The therapist thought to himself that this hierarchical construction of their relationship might be where Fred and Luke were stuck. He began to wonder simultaneously why their disagreements often deteriorated into shouting matches. Threatening to end a relationship, a tactic that Fred seemed to use as their arguments escalated, can be a power maneuver. Such tactics are often invoked when one partner is so sensitive to the other that he has difficulty holding onto the "I"—his own individuality—as he becomes a "we" with his partner. However, such a threat is a maneuver that is extremely destructive to the relationship, forcing the couple repeatedly to detach from each other psychologically. In fact, we find that threat to be so destructive that we make a contract with couples in treatment to not use any threat of breakup in arguments.

The therapist said to this couple: "Together we will see if you can find a more constructive way to feel more in control and less threatened when you have a disagreement. Then you won't have to use tactics that potentially destroy the relationship when you have a disagreement." Language is one way we construct our reality. The therapist wanted to communicate to the couple that the use of the "breakup" word was not only destructive but destabilizing for their relationship. Separating should not be the first option for any couple confronted with differences.

The therapist continued to explore with both partners what might happen next when Fred made good on his threat to end the relationship. Often Fred would move back to his former apartment and sleep on the sofa for a few days (possible further evidence of his tenuous commitment and trust in their relationship). Soon he would realize that he couldn't live without Luke and would then move back in. The therapist asked if their arguments ever deteriorated from verbal abuse into physical violence, and both men said Fred occasionally slammed doors but that they had never physically hurt each other. Fred was much larger than his slight partner, and the therapist wondered aloud if Luke ever felt intimidated. Luke nodded agreement that he often got scared when they argued but that he was unwilling to "back down." Then Luke said something the therapist felt continued to confirm his hypothesis of a teacher–student complementary relationship. He said, "I often find myself anxious when we're at home together because I feel that I'll do something wrong and set Fred off."

It was at this point in the first session that the therapist felt he had joined sufficiently with the couple and that he had enough information to create an initial map of their relationship. He now wanted to test his hypothesis by creating an enactment. It is often helpful if a therapist stands up in the session and invites one member of the couple to move to another place in order to face his partner. The therapist can simply say, "In family treatment, we do all kinds of strange things. Please move over here so you can see your partner better." The partner invariably consents. The therapist is making a transition in the session from a state that is more social to one that is more attuned to therapeutic interaction. The therapist's move dramatizes this transition and sets the stage. Moving Luke off the sofa where the couple had been seated and into a chair also elevated him in the session. As Fred appeared to have the dominant voice in their relationship, the therapist may have been already anticipating how he would unbalance this construction as he staged their first enactment.

As we noted earlier, when staging an enactment, the therapist needs to help the couple to focus on a specific topic. Often the couple will choose a general area of conflict in their relationship. "We never agree about anything" is potentially useful information but may not be specific enough for the partner to respond to. (Also, such general statement can come across as a form of character assassination or can strike the criticized partner as indicating that their situation is hopeless. It is more constructive and helpful for the couple to problem solve by choosing to discuss a *specific* incident when they have got stuck in the past or are currently in a disagreement.)

As the therapist got Luke to move to the chair opposite Fred, he asked the couple to think of a time recently when they got into an argument that seemed irresolvable. They both thought of the same incident that had occurred over the weekend and had the potential to have deteriorated into a shouting match and stand-off. Luke said that he had been slicing up vegetables for a dip they were going to serve for their dinner guests. Fred walked into the kitchen and told Luke that he was slicing the vegetables too thick.

The therapist now had specific material to stage an enactment. Rather than listen to how the couple said they interacted, through the enactment the therapist would have an opportunity to *experience* the couple's interpersonal dynamics. He asked the two men to talk about this specific incident, sensing that in the details of this incident he might observe what was problematic in the relationship that they had constructed. As the enactment began, Fred immediately spoke to Luke in an authoritarian voice, telling him that crudités needed to be bite-sized. At one point in his lecture, he shook his finger at Luke to emphasize his point. Luke turned to the therapist and in a pleading voice said, "I'm not real good in the kitchen." This pull for triangulation, to induct the therapist into the couple's dynamic, is common (Bowen, 1978). Either to defuse the tension or perhaps to rescue himself, Luke was trying to bring the therapist into their argument. The therapist needed to stand firm and not allow himself to become an intermediary in their disagreement. He simply but firmly said, "Please, talk to your partner." Often it will take several attempts or even sessions for a therapist to educate a couple to the culture of structural therapy. Eventually they will realize that the therapist is not going to rescue them and they need to problem solve with each other.

Luke stared at the therapist helplessly and then turned back to Fred. Luke initially began to talk to Fred in a pleading voice. "You know I don't pay attention to details. What difference does it make if the vegetables are one bite or two-bite size?" Fred responded in a paternal voice, "People don't want to get the dip all over themselves. It's neater when you slice thin." This interaction continued between them for several minutes. Fred continued to lecture, and Luke continued to dispute his suggestions, gradually raising his voice. As Luke became more assertive, Fred glared at him and turned pale. It was obvious that no resolution would come out of this disagreement.

The therapist said to them, "Luke, it seems that you are still caught in a student–teacher relationship from your training days—only you're no longer being a cooperative student. Perhaps being a student no longer serves either of you. Fred, you seem determined to teach Luke your way of slicing vegetables. Luke, perhaps you don't need Fred to be your teacher anymore, and you don't know how to tell him." The language the therapist used here highlighted the complementary roles in their relationship and the pas de deux that they were engaged in, and anticipated the unbalancing that would occur later in treatment.

It always is an interesting dynamic in the construction of any couple's relationship when one of the partners takes on a student role. Eventually the student is going to experience growing pains and want to demonstrate his competency. The new behavior challenges the implicit contract that the couple has constructed as to who is the leader and who is the follower. Unless a couple is flexible and able to negotiate new roles, a crisis will occur as they struggle to change the rules of their relationship.

Luke was rebelling from his student role, and Fred appeared to feel threatened by this role expansion on his partner's part. Fred initially tried to overpower Luke psychologically and, failing to do that, he withdrew. Fred's distancing only exacerbated the circular dynamic as Luke became more anxious and insecure about their relationship. The more anxious he became, the more assertive Luke was in demanding an equal voice. Couple treatment would need to provide them with the space to experiment with new ways of taking turns in leader and follower roles.

DON AND GERRY REVISITED

In Chapter 4 we talked about joining with Don and Gerry, a couple in their early 40s. Gerry had brought Don into treatment because Don had recently started going to clubs and using illicit drugs such as Ecstasy. Gerry was concerned that Don's behavior might not only harm his health but also get him into trouble with the law. The therapist felt concerned that his drug use would also destabilize their relationship. Early in treatment the therapist was aware that he felt a strong pull to become a parent and counsel Don into behaving more responsibly.

The therapist had been in a dilemma about how to respond to Don's use of drugs. He found himself pulled to assume the role of educator—identical to Gerry's role with Don. While we acknowledge that Don's behavior was self-destructive, the novelty of the structural family therapist's role is to introduce a focus on the systemic meaning of the behavior, and thereby to help Don and Gerry take responsibility for their lives. However, the therapist could not ignore Don's substance abuse. He was organized by his work with other gay men who had become clinically depressed after repeated uses of recreational drugs. The therapist felt the need to make a judgment call as to the seriousness of Don's drug use. He felt it would be irresponsible because of the potential consequences if he did not do some psychoeducation about the potential long-term deleterious effects of recreational drugs. This pull to become an educator and a cop in session is not the family therapist's best use of himself but one that a therapist can feel compelled to take up. The danger in taking up the role of the educator and cop for the system is that the therapist starts to do the work of the couple.

As he joined with the couple, the therapist began to think, "Why this behavior, and why now in their relationship?" The therapist hypothesized that the couple might be at a transition phase in their relationship when Don wanted more closeness with Gerry but was at a loss as to how to acknowledge and express this need. Early in treatment Gerry had expressed a commitment to continue to parent his adolescent son. What was confusing to the therapist was that Gerry appeared to be emotionally more invested in his relationship with his son's mother than with Don. Don appeared to be the third wheel in this arrangement and was possibly rebelling against this arrangement with self-destructive behavior. The therapist knew that simply making an interpretation would not necessarily produce change. He needed to stage an enactment that would give him and the couple a window to observe their style of relating to each other. He needed to discover what dynamics in their relationship were maintaining Don's rebellious behavior.

The therapist asked Don to sit in a chair opposite his partner. As he set up the enactment, the therapist said he wasn't sure how this might have happened but he thought that Don was lonely. The therapist then invited the two men to talk with each other about how they could be more connected. Gerry smiled confidently at the therapist and began to tell him that all he ever wanted was to be in a loving relationship with Don but he was baffled by Don's irresponsible behavior. The therapist resisted the invitation to diffuse their tension and instead said, "Talk to your partner. Somehow he doesn't get your concern." Gerry turned to Don and said he was amazed and bewildered by his club attendance. He said, "You're endangering your health, and you could get into trouble with the law for using drugs." He elaborated on his concerns with a lecture to Don on the legal implications of his possession of Ecstasy. Gerry expressed his worries in a polite manner, more like a school principal speaking to an errant pupil. Don remained silent and glared at his partner. When the therapist encouraged Don to respond, he said curtly, "If you don't like it, you can go back to your wife. I'm over 40 now. I intend to enjoy my life."

The therapist again felt conflicted. Gerry's argument was logical and his concerns were legitimate. But if the therapist intervened to reinforce Gerry's worries, he once again would risk getting caught in problem solving over the couple's predicament. He would not have introduced any systemic meaning to the story, and he would have accepted and reinforced Gerry's narrow definition of their problem. According to Gerry, Don was acting like a rebellious adolescent, and the message from Gerry was that he wanted the therapist to reprimand him.

If the therapist accepted this narrow definition of their problem, he too would be defeated. He would have bought the couple's story, and nothing would have changed. Couples have spent many years constructing their relationship, producing a rigid story that has more potency than any therapist's ability to problem solve. The therapist must enter the couple's system in some manner that not only interrupts their story but also gives them an opportunity to understand how the behaviors that they complain about are a symptom of how they interact.

The therapist had two obvious choices of interventions here. He might ask Gerry, "How have you made your partner so bored he needs to hit the clubs to find excitement in his life?" Another possibility would be for the therapist to ask Don something totally nonlinear, such as "Do you think Gerry will ever divorce his wife and marry you?" In either case the therapist needs to introduce novelty by making a choice not to support the couple's story that Don is the patient in this scenario. If the therapist wanted to further challenge the way the couple were interacting, he would need to support Don in the session so that he had more of a voice.

It appeared that up until now Don was acting out his feelings in the role of a rebellious teenager rather than voicing his dissatisfactions. The therapist was aware of his feeling that Don's behavior might be motivated by loneliness. The problem appeared to be that Don's behavior was having the undesirable effect of driving Gerry toward his wife. As he staged an enactment, he wanted to create a space for Don to talk with Gerry in a way that might engage Gerry.

Notice here that the therapist is already working on at least two levels. On one level he is creating intensity through the enactments to ascertain if the couple can remain proximal while disagreeing. Simultaneously he is beginning to unbalance the couple's repetitive dance by supporting Don in getting out of the role of the identified patient. "Don," the therapist said, "tell Gerry why you're so angry at him."

Instead of talking to Gerry, Don began to talk with the therapist. He began talking slowly but quickly gained momentum. He said Gerry had never divorced his wife. In fact, not only were they not divorced but they still owned joint properties. Furthermore, when the men vaca-tioned together, Gerry often invited his wife and their son to join them. For a moment, the therapist became totally caught up in Don's plight and forgot the request that he had made for the couple to interact. This was new and important information that Don was revealing. Don was both articulate and forceful as he listed his complaints.

The therapist asked how the experience of having Gerry's wife on their vacation had affected Don's vacation time with Gerry. Don said he was initially fine with the arrangement but that, as time went on, he felt resentful. Early on in their relationship, he wanted them to have a home together large enough for the son to visit. During the past year he had come to the conclusion that Gerry would never listen to his wishes, and he had given up trying. Ending the session for that day, the therapist wondered aloud whether Don's partying might be his last attempt to save the relationship.

The therapist thought between sessions how quickly he had aban-doned the enactment and been seduced into siding with Don after ini-tially experiencing a pull to take up Gerry's role in attempting to stop Don's drug use. The therapist realized he would have to be careful with this couple so that he didn't become triangulated with one partner against the other.

During the next session the therapist encouraged Don to talk directly with Gerry. Don quickly found his voice. He blasted Gerry for the ways that he felt neglected during the past several years of their rela-tionship. He talked more about the vacations, complaining that Gerry had spent more time with his wife and son than he had with him. He lambasted him for never divorcing or even severing his ties with his wife so that he and Gerry could be freer to make their own home. Gerry responded defensively, saying that he was going to get a divorce but he was waiting for the real estate market to peak, so that he could realize the maximum profit on the sale of their jointly owned property.

Don interrupted by saying, "That's bullshit. We have more than enough money." Don continued to pour out his anger as Gerry stopped talking and eventually shut down. At this point the therapist had ob-served enough of their dance.

The therapist said, "Don, keep talking, but you may want to see if you can find ways to revive Gerry. I think you've knocked him out with your bat." Then, turning to Gerry, he said, "Gerry, is this when you turn toward your wife, to be resuscitated?" The enactment had illuminated their circular dance as both men initially frowned and then laughed in recognition of their predictable pattern.

THE CONTINUED SAGA
OF THE CARETAKER AND HIS PATIENT

Ernie and James were the couple we introduced in the preceding chapter who disagreed over opening up their relationship to multiple sexual partners. The therapist initially acknowledged their differences and said he would return to the problem but he would first like to know them better as a couple. As the therapist took a history of their relationship, he discovered that they had constructed a relationship with what appeared to be extreme disparity in their levels of functioning. James was holding down two jobs as the couple struggled to make ends meet. James supported Ernie's unemployed status and, similar to Ernie's father, felt that Ernie shouldn't have to struggle hard in earning a living. When the therapist asked Ernie if he was medically unable to work after his accident, James responded for him by saying that Ernie needed to continue to rest.

During the early stages of treatment, when the therapist encouraged the two men to discuss their precarious financial arrangements, Ernie deferred to James's decisions about the allocation of their resources. It became clear to the therapist that James did the lion's share of the work in their relationship, and the therapist speculated that James made most of the executive decisions. Ernie's role appeared to be that of an ungrateful student. He would complain and whine, but he had no voice of consequence in their relationship. When the therapist asked them to discuss possible solutions to their debt problem, James patiently explained to Ernie that he needed to be more frugal in his spending. Not only was James the primary provider, but also he spoke to Ernie as though he alone was the possessor of knowledge in their relationship.

During one session an enactment occurred between the couple in which Ernie was reduced to the role of a rebellious teenager. James told Ernie, "Stop eating out so much; we could save a lot of money if you stopped insisting we eat at restaurants." Ernie snapped back at him, "I'm bored with the food we eat." Initially the therapist thought James's request quite rational and Ernie's response to be that of a spoiled child.

But he continued to observe the two, knowing that if he intervened he would be caught up in the content of their argument. The therapist observed James' posture in the session, sitting tall with one foot under him and his hands folded in his lap while Ernie continued gesturing with his hands as he argued without much conviction.

The therapist knew he needed to intervene at the process level of their relationship to effectively reflect their hierarchically constructed relationship. He introduced a nonlinear frame. The therapist first spoke to Ernie: "It's becoming clearer to me why you might want to open up your relationship, Ernie. James has become your guru as well as your caretaker. You can't have sex with your guru." Then, before Ernie could respond, he turned to James. "James, how did you get in such an elevated position?" Though it was early in the couple's treatment, the metaphor of the guru and his student created by the therapist highlighted the skewed dynamic of their relationship.

The therapist's introduction of the "guru–student" metaphor temporarily interrupted the partners' dance, but they quickly regained their equilibrium. The therapist decided to take another tact by choosing to help the couple focus on issues where Ernie might gain a more competent role in their relationship. For instance, in one session the therapist encouraged Ernie to become more proactive in decision making about the allocation of their resources. He encouraged the two men in session to create a budget and intentionally gave Ernie the role of bookkeeper. However, James continued to infantalize Ernie. James would nod in agreement as Ernie spoke, but it was clear to the therapist that he was merely placating Ernie, not engaging him. Ernie continued to participate in this predictable dance by abdicating his position as a responsible partner. Homework tasks were equally inefficacious. Ernie would say he would start looking for employment, but by the next session nothing would have happened. He was neither contributing to the family resources nor adhering to the day-to-day budgeting plans they had agreed to in session. At one point he said to James, "You're right. You're always right. I'm just a total fuckup."

The couple continued to remain stuck, with Ernie in the underfunctioning role of the "patient/ student" and James in the role of "caretaker/guru." The therapist speculated that Ernie had outgrown this arrangement but that James, though poor, was finding some sort of reward in his role as caretaker/guru. Ernie's growing pains challenged the status quo. Their system was rigid and insufficiently flexible to accommodate Ernie's desire to grow up. The therapist hypothesized to himself that Ernie's challenge to James to open their relationship was his attempt to find his own voice.

The therapist continued to be caught in the role of coach, as he urged Ernie to be more financially resourceful. However, the role of coach, though potentially helpful, is often not an effective one in altering a couple's interpersonal dynamics.

At the beginning of the fourth session, the couple literally burst into the therapist's office, energized. Ernie, rather than slouching, sat up in his chair and began by saying that they had engaged in a fight. The therapist was surprised, as Ernie and James had previously carefully avoided any conflict. "The fight" had consisted of Ernie shoving James and hitting him in the head with a pillow. Both men were surprised at the intensity of emotion they had experienced. Interestingly, Ernie, for the first time since treatment had begun, did not appear depressed. He was alive and animated in the session. James too was different. He appeared less self-satisfied, and his body language had changed. Rather than sitting in a half-lotus position, he faced Ernie and was more receptive to what his partner had to say.

The two men used the next couple of sessions to strategize cooperatively over possible solutions to their financial problems. The therapist supported this new behavior and simultaneously managed to stay out of the role of coach as he observed them collaborating. Ernie began to take a much more active role in devising solutions regarding food budgeting and other household expenses. James listened to his partner's suggestions and concurred with many of them.

During the seventh session Ernie and James were more affectionate than they had been earlier, at one point even holding hands with each other. They told the therapist that they had been sexually intimate with each other for the first time in several months. Both men felt more hopeful about their relationship.

Ernie then announced to James and the therapist that he had obtained an office-temp job. James was speechless as Ernie told him the news. As the therapist encouraged the two men to talk with each other about the details of Ernie's job, he noticed that James was elated over this turn of events. Ernie said he wanted to be more of a contributor to their relationship and for them to become more financially solvent as a couple. The therapist was delighted for them, got up out of his chair, and shook hands with each of them to underscore the significance of this new behavior.

After the men got over the excitement of discussing Ernie's news, James did something new and unexpected. He began to disclose to Ernie the details of a problem that he was experiencing with his employer. Ernie listened and gave him suggestions as to how he might resolve the misunderstanding with his boss. The therapist knew he needed to further highlight this new behavior. He asked James to tell Ernie how he had experienced his newly supportive partner. The therapist was careful in his choice of words, feeling James appreciated being out of the role of caretaker and knowing James would need to reinforce this new dynamic. James told Ernie he was comforted by his suggestions and appreciated Ernie being able to help him. Ernie beamed with pleasure. These enactments had spontaneously led the couple into an unbalancing of old behaviors and expansion to new roles—James for the first time was leaning on Ernie for support and caretaking.

During the ninth session the couple elaborated on the details of Ernie's financial dependency on his family. Ernie elaborated to the therapist why he hid from his parents the nature of his relationship with James. Both men said they feared that Ernie's parents would withhold money if they thought it was primarily used to support them as a couple.

This level of secrecy is something that we rarely see in our work with heterosexual couples, but it is not uncommon for gay couples. The secrecy usually occurs because of one or both men's fear of their parents' reprisals or disapproval of their relationship. The therapist was intrigued by this arrangement and wondered aloud in session what price the couple might be paying for this arrangement. Both men responded simultaneously: the price was to remain asexual in the eyes of Ernie's parents. Although out to his family since high school, Ernie had remained asexual. He had never introduced any boyfriend to his parents, nor had he ever suggested to them that he was sexually active with men. This sounded to the therapist like a version of the "don't ask, don't tell" U.S. armed forces policy toward gays that exacts such an enormous penalty on the self-esteem of gay men. Perhaps Ernie's parents were supportive of this homophobia.

The therapist was in a bind at this point. If the couple had been heterosexual and keeping their relationship secret from their families, the therapist would have highlighted the dynamic, as such secrecy could negatively impact on their continuing to maintain a long-term stable relationship. Yet, the therapist needed to be respectful of the culture of Ernie's family. James was cut off from his own family. Ernie's family offered both men a family support system. James spoke of having a warm relationship with Ernie's father. The therapist did not want to destroy the healthy aspects of this relationship.

The therapist also thought about Ernie's stage of gay identity development. Although he had disclosed his same-sex attraction to his parents and reported being comfortable with his gayness since high school, could he have nonetheless internalized our culture's taboo against homosexuality and feel ashamed to reveal the sexual/romantic relationship he had with James to his parents?

As the therapist explored their relationship with their families, Ernie and James talked about spending major family holidays with Ernie's parents. On these occasions, the men slept in Ernie's childhood bedroom. The men jokingly told stories about how Ernie's mother would enter their bedroom without knocking on their door. The men never objected and continued to pass as roommates. The therapist decided to challenge the men's arrangement, as he expressed his concern for them as a couple. "Ernie's financial umbilical cord," he said, "might be exacting great costs on your collective well-being."

The men on many levels were struggling to become a couple. Ernie's desire to renegotiate the rules of their relationship threatened an already precarious identity as a couple. Although they had not returned to the topic of an open relationship since the first session, the therapist wondered aloud if opening the relationship might not be less threatening than confronting the parents' behavior that seemed to keep Ernie in a childlike status. Both men's behavior contributed to this dependent relationship, as James supported Ernie's secretiveness and colluded with the system's denial of their couplehood. As the session ended, the therapist wasn't sure how or if they would resolve this dilemma and potential threat to their couplehood.

THE DANCE OF THE TWO BULLS

As a final example of the power of enactments to reveal interpersonal behavioral patterns, we will describe a couple in treatment for 20 sessions. The therapist had been unable to discover what dynamics maintained where the couple was stuck until he sought out a consultation with a senior colleague and inadvertently introduced novelty into a session. During the playback of a videotaped session, both the therapist and the couple discovered the many ways that homophobia had organized their behavior to preclude intimacy.

In their mid-30s, Paul and David were each brokers in highly successful real estate firms. In the first session when the therapist had asked them why they had sought out therapy, each man said that they had unresolvable arguments that wore each of them down. Paul felt so alienated by these arguments that he was seriously considering ending the relationship. David seemed equally discouraged, but he was not ready to separate.

The therapist asked David and Paul if each could give him an example of what they argued about, and both men related recent incidents. Paul told of a incident when David was in the kitchen preparing a gourmet dinner and David would not permit him to enter the room. David spoke angrily of an incident when he was playing an electronic game of chess and Paul continually leaned over his shoulder and told him what moves to make.

Both men appeared to be incensed by the other's intrusiveness. Initially David and Paul seemed totally unable to spare any energy in avoiding a verbal contest to prove that the other was wrong. Each postured and bellowed as they swiped at each other with their grievances. Paul's complaint was that David was "too clinging." Before the therapist could ask David to express what he would like to improve in his relationship with Paul, David retaliated in kind, calling Paul "a control freak." Eventually, as they grew tired of these endless battles, Paul would shut down and David would turn to the therapist to problem solve. The therapist experienced their dynamics as a tidal wave, knocking him off balance. He liked each man individually, but as a couple their late-in-the-day sessions were toxic and wore him down. Alternatively, he found himself daydreaming in sessions, an unusual experience for him and one that should have alerted him to his need for a consultation, himself.

Early during treatment the therapist reflected that it was clear that both partners were miserable and appeared to have great difficulty in resolving their differences. And then he said they would return to this issue of what appeared to be a constant sparring contest where no one was winning. As he made the transition to history-taking, he wondered aloud what would happen if each put down the boxing gloves, for a change.

Their history as a couple reflected two men who cared a great deal for each other as they built their life together. Paul said that he had met David 5 years ago, soon after David had moved to New York from the rural South. At that time David was waiting on tables in Greenwich Village, trying to get established as a film editor. David talked about his economic struggle as an artist with no clear career path on his horizon. Paul said he was already established as a realtor and was positioned to make large sums of money in a booming commercial real estate market. He encouraged David to study for his real estate license, and then he helped him set up his own small firm. For the first couple of years both men thrived under this arrangement. The complementary roles initially constructed by this couple seemed clear: Paul was the mentor and David took up the role of protégé. The therapist would need to test his hypothesis with an enactment. The map (Figure 5.1), if valid, suggests the course of treatment to create greater parity in the men's relationship.

The structural therapist thought this arrangement had probably served Paul and David well through the "honeymoon" phase of their relationship. He speculated that, as David matured, he would at some point chafe in his one-down position as protégé. This kind of inequity is a common dynamic for couples, and often a crisis is precipitated when the protégé rebels. Couples frequently come into treatment at this transitional phase in their relationship as they attempt to renegotiate roles. For heterosexual couples with children, the crisis may occur when the "empty nest" syndrome occurs in their life cycle and Mom wants to reinvest her energies in a new career. Or, if the couple is a two-career family, and one of the partner's career suddenly takes off, the shift

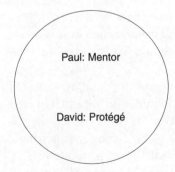

FIGURE 5.1. Structural map for Paul and David.

in earning power can challenge the relationship. Similarly, age differences in relationships can initially be complementary, and later a source of stress as the younger partner grows up. The therapist initially thought that David's career success and increased earning power might be a factor threatening the roles that this couple had constructed.

During history taking in the joining phase, the therapist had learned that Paul and David each came from a very different background from the other. Paul was raised in an affluent urban Jewish-Italian family, and David grew up in a poor rural southern WASP community. Their differences had complemented one another as Paul introduced David to New York City. Early in their courtship, Paul's knowledge of the city and relatively high income enabled them to take advantage of the city's culture. Both men had many similar interests in the arts. They enjoyed the downtown music scene and Off Off-Broadway theater. They had become active in the gay rights movement and in various political fund-raising events. The men talked enthusiastically about having created a commitment ceremony 2 years into their relationship and legalizing their relationship by registering as domestic partners at City Hall. They were out to their families, and both families and friends had participated in their commitment ritual.

The therapeutic value to gay couples of creating their own rituals and ceremonies should not be overlooked during the history-taking phase of treatment. For couples isolated from the majority culture, rituals such as commitment ceremonies not only formalize same-sex unions but also are a vehicle for them to publicly acknowledge their commitment. Such rituals bring together a community to witness the couple's commitment to each other and to acknowledge the couple's need for the support of their extended family.

David and Paul also talked appreciatively about the cultural differences distinguishing urban Jewish from rural WASP influences that existed between their families when they alternated holidays. They had an active social life and talked about sharing many friends in common, both gay and straight individuals and couples. This couple had many strengths and a strong foundation on which to build a life together.

After the therapist had taken a history of their relationship, he said they appeared to be stuck in a critical stage of the couple's relationship as they struggled to redefine their roles. He wasn't sure what the prize was for the victor, but the verbal sparring that they continually engaged in appeared to cause both of them a lot of pain. They agreed with him, but the intervention that labeled their dance for what it was did nothing to illuminate or unbalance the dynamic.

The therapist had hit the wall. During repeated enactments, each man appeared committed to a desire to be the dominator of the other. They continued to battle during sessions over seemingly trivial issues— who takes the shirts to the laundry, who cleans up the apartment, where they would spend their vacation (the list of subjects on which they could disagree seemed endless). Their battles were like Chinese water torture for the therapist.

The therapist asked David and Paul for examples of exceptions: were there any occasions when they were able to collaborate? Paul quickly responded with his example of collaboration. Paul said the purchase of their apartment had been a collaborative experience for him. However, when the therapist asked if they had joint ownership, Paul said it was his money that had been used to purchase the apartment and the deed to the apartment was in his name. His example of collaboration was actually a unilateral decision with minimal input from David. When it came to decorating the apartment, their efforts at collaboration broke down as David struggled to assert control.

During these enactments, both men were articulate in their arguments, organizing their conversations like two attorneys going into litigation. They frequently interrupted each other. Speaking in paragraphs, rarely did they leave space for contemplation or for the other to organize his thoughts. Each would cut the other off in mid-sentence.

The therapist continued to summarize the dynamics at work in ways that reflected the couple's circular arguments. The couple would momentarily pause as they allowed the therapist to speak and then continue with their struggle as if nothing had been said. Unable to interrupt these highly reactive and destructive patterns, the therapist made a decision to coach the couple in basic listener–speaker exercises (Gottman, Notarius, Gonso, & Markman, 1976). These exercises are often effective for highly conflicted couples, as they force the partners to slow down their verbal exchanges. The exercises encourage each partner to speak concisely and to listen attentively. They are often helpful for argumentative couples who are caught up in power struggles and unable to hear each other's point of view. The exercises force the partners to become better listeners as each learns to become more reflective and observant of his communication style.

David and Paul required little coaching and were readily able to paraphrase accurately what the other had said. With the therapist's coaching, they were able to identify feelings activated by the other's behaviors and to communicate their feelings to each other within the structure of the exercise. However, when the therapist asked them to practice the speaker–listener exercises at home using low-conflict topics to reinforce the skills that they had learned in sessions, they would end up reporting during the following session that the practice periods had been unmitigated disasters. Apparently, at home neither had the patience to listen to the other. Paul would tell David to hurry up his story and speak faster. David became furious as he listened to the content of Paul's communication and would interrupt. While they were good students in the therapist's office, they were miserable students at home.

The men were quick to defend themselves. Each seemed most comfortable expressing anger, and neither man appeared willing to express his more vulnerable feelings. Nothing the therapist did seemed to interrupt their destructive communication patterns. The therapist felt like a failure in session and ended each session feeling frustrated and hopeless.

We view the continual expression of anger in couple's treatment as a defensive emotion that one or both partners use to protect their more vulnerable core selves. While the expression of anger can be effective when it leads to the authentic expression of a partner's viewpoint and doesn't denigrate the other, to vent anger for anger's sake with no goal of therapeutic change is both destructive and self-indulgent. A goal of treatment for many male couples is to create an environ where the men feel safe to explore any shame that they may have around their needs for affection and intimacy in their relationship. This level of work is essential in the treatment of gay men, who frequently are inexperienced and fearful of expressing needs for softness and affection with another man.

At this stage of the treatment, it appeared that the male therapist, also gay, was caught in a coaching mode of treatment that may have blinded him to the couple's lack of comfort with intimacy. He continued to introduce exercises that he hoped might be helpful to illuminate where they were stuck. The other possibility was that the male therapist was caught in his own discomfort with male intimacy. In either case, he needed to consult with a colleague.

MONDAY MORNING QUARTERBACKS:
THE BENEFITS OF SUPERVISION AND VIDEOTAPES

Prior to his planned consultation with a senior colleague, the therapist had a scheduled session with the couple during which he had decided to try family sculpting exercises (Duhl, Kantor, & Duhl, 1973). These exercises are often effective with intellectualized families, where the cultural norm is to avoid the expression of feelings. The exercises often will get people out of their heads and into their feelings. Feelings are often easier to express nonverbally. For families with children the exercises can be a lot of fun, because the children have an opportunity to tell their parents what to do, as each person in the family takes a turn at being the sculptor. As this is a nonverbal exercise, the therapist may have hoped he was introducing novelty and an opportunity for David and Paul to express their more tender feelings.

The task of this exercise is for each member of the family to nonverbally create a visual sculpture that is an expression of the dynamics of their family as they experience them. Initially, the sculptor physically places each member of the family in a pose that expresses that individual's role or emotional style in the family. Once he has positioned everyone in a pose that expresses their role in the family, the sculptor then places himself into the sculpture as he experiences himself in relation to the others. The therapist needs to coach the sculptor to remember not to talk, as most family members will want to talk to one another as they are sculpting. Talking at this point in the exercise is forbidden, however, as it dilutes the emotional experience.

Once the sculptor has created the sculpture, the therapist asks them to freeze in their positions. The therapist then asks each person to notice what it feels like to be in this sculpture. There is still no talking permitted by anyone other than the therapist.

It's often helpful if the therapist gets up at this point and circles the sculpture to fully see how the sculptor has placed each person. If the exercise is effective, the sculptor will have created a visual representation of how he experiences the dynamics of his family system. At this point the therapist asks the sculptor to describe his creation. The therapist then asks each family member to describe what it feels like to be a part of the sculpture.

Many families are highly creative in this process and create sculptures that will eventually lead to more flexible roles in their relationships. For instance, an adolescent once created a sculpture of his family in which each member of the family was walking in circles totally disconnected visually and physically from one another. After he had each member of the family placed exactly as he related to them, he then darted in and out of the circle they were walking in, frantically waving as he attempted to get his parent's attention or to connect with his younger siblings. His attempts were pointless, as he had each of them positioned so that their eyes were averted, either looking at the floor or up at the ceiling. When asked to describe the sculpture, the adolescent talked about his family's seeming so unrelated, each person living in his or her own world.

His family had come into treatment after his mother had been discharged from a physical rehabilitation center following a nearly fatal accident. The mother was hospitalized for several months on life-support systems, but no one in the family would talk about the tragedy of what had happened to this woman and the extraordinary role shifts that needed to occur in response to her disability. The sculpting exercise gave them the opportunity to start to put into words the complexity of feelings that had been repressed during her hospitalization and to begin to explore how each of them could take up new roles in the family.

In the case of David and Paul, each man sculpted representations of their relationship that expressed needs for closeness but at different levels. Paul's sculpture depicted David as standing behind him, one arm around his waist, as Paul stretched both arms out in an opposite direction. When asked to describe his sculpture, Paul said that he was struggling to get out of David's grip, but that David wouldn't let him go. As they held the positions that Paul had sculpted, the therapist asked each man to describe what it felt like to be in the sculpture. David began to cry as he described the frustration he experienced trying to hold onto Paul. Paul said he felt exhausted from the tug-of-war sculpture that he had created with David.

David sculpted a representation of their relationship that was both similar to and quite different from Paul's. Paul was still standing with his arms extended in an opposite direction from David, but Paul's back was against David's, and David's arms were extended too. David had placed each of them as listing in opposite directions. When asked to describe his sculpture, David said that the forms represented the two men searching for each other but unable to see or support the other. David said he felt off-balance and disconnected from his partner. Paul reported feeling lonely and frustrated. What was novel for the men, and hopeful for the therapist, was that each was able to describe feelings other than anger that were evoked in the sculpture.

The next phase in the exercise, paralleling the unbalancing phase of structural therapy, is for each member of the family to have an opportunity to create a representational configuration of how he would like to relate to members of his family. This is another version of a "magic wand" exercise. The therapist might say, "If you could fast forward the therapy to termination, could you sculpt how you would like to relate to your family?" Often families really enjoy this phase of the sculpting, as it allows them to become more creative and hopeful.

Paul and David were no exception, as they immediately started to laugh and became much more playful while each took a turn in creating his "ideal sculpture." Paul made a sculpture in which each man stood side by side, holding hands. He placed their heads so that they were looking in slightly different directions. When asked to describe what he had depicted, he said the sculpture represented them going about their daily work, connected but free to explore the world. The therapist asked them to describe how it felt to be in these positions, and each man had dramatically different responses. Paul said that he felt liberated and no longer in a tug-of-war. David, however, felt somewhat disconnected from his partner and continued to feel sad and lonely.

David then created his ideal of the relationship. In this sculpture, David seated himself on the office sofa and had Paul seated beside him. He then put his arms around Paul's shoulders. David described the sculpture as the two men living together in harmony without any conflict between them. Paul responded dramatically to this sculpture and said that he felt claustrophobic. David, not surprisingly, said that he felt more secure in this position. What may be obvious is that, although the partners depicted different comfort levels for closeness in their sculptures, each showed a similar need for greater connectedness in their relationship.

Sculpting is an opportunity for couples and families to begin to understand how their interpersonal needs differ. Their complementary styles will often become more explicit as the roles in the family system become evident through the sculpture. Often, insights and alternative styles to their rigidified patterns of behavior will become apparent as each person creates his "ideal sculpture."

However, in David and Paul's case, they used the exercise as one more way to beat each other up. David accused Paul of wanting to control him, and Paul countered with an attack on David's emotional immaturity. The therapist was at a loss as to how he might get the couple to become more observant of the dance that they were doing that precluded closeness. Before their next session, he did consult with a senior colleague. Together they watched the video of the previous sculpting session to see if they might get some insight into the couple's struggle.

Watching the video recording of a family therapy session has many benefits for a therapist. It's the equivalent of "Monday morning quarterbacking." A therapist has an opportunity to observe the session free of the emotional pulls that can induct him into a family's system. Viewing a videotape gives a therapist the freedom to explore alternative interventions that might help him to unbalance a family system's dynamic in the subsequent session. A therapist also has the luxury of discussing the case with a colleague who can help him deconstruct the session and expand his conceptualization of the case. Another benefit of videotaping sessions is that a therapist can choose to show segments of the session to the couple for help in understanding what was going on.

Watching this video of Paul and David's sculpting session, both the therapist and the consultant were perplexed by the couple's responses. Rather than using the exercise as an opportunity to explore how they had constructed a relationship that seemed not to meet each of their needs for closeness, they used it as yet another weapon for beating each other up. In watching the tape, both the consultant and the therapist were moved as each of the men depicted how he would like to be more connected to his partner. While each man had different needs for affiliation, they both indicated a desire to be more intimate. This is information that the therapist might use as leverage to explore what each man needed to do for his partner to create more intimacy. However, the exercise itself had proved ineffective in creating new behavior for this couple.

The heterosexual male consultant asked the gay male therapist many questions. He was interested in knowing if this couple knew how to soothe each other. Had one taught the other how he would like to be comforted? They appeared agitated in the session, and he wondered if their verbal sparring wasn't a smoke screen that obscured their needs for softness and tenderness. The therapist was unable to answer the consultant's questions. These were areas he had failed to explore with David and Paul.

The therapist was confused as to how he would proceed with the couple. With the concurrence of the consultant, he decided to show the couple the videotape of their sculpting session. Before showing them the sculpting exercise tape, the therapist simply said, "Guys, I'm stuck. Help me to understand what is going on in this session."

Their responses were totally unexpected and gave new meaning to the destructiveness of homophobia.

The men were mortified watching the videotape of their sculpting session. Besides the usual embarrassment that all of us experience when we initially see and hear ourselves on tape, they also laughed as they both acknowledged the accuracy of the sculptures. Although neither man was prone to self-reflection, they both concurred with the therapist's interpretation that they were engaged in a power struggle. But the therapist could never have predicted what they revealed next.

On the videotape, after each man sculpted his version of his ideal relationship and gave feedback, they both sat down on the sofa in the therapist's office. Apparently exhausted, David momentarily leaned into Paul as Paul put his arms around David and gave him a kiss on the forehead. As they viewed this sequence of the tape, both men groaned, "Yuck!" Thinking that the men were having a delayed response to seeing themselves caught in another squabble, the therapist stopped the tape. He asked them to elaborate on their joint "Yuck!"

Each of the men began to describe how silly and uncomfortable he felt observing each other acting so "effeminate" on the video. The therapist was at a loss as to what they were referring to and asked them to elaborate. David said that they had always prided themselves in not appearing as "Chelsea boys," a reference to a stereotype of buffed gay men who openly express their queerness. Both men agreed that they were offended by gay men who showed affection toward one another in public.

The enactments that the therapist had observed suddenly became clearer with the revelation of this material. Although caught in a power struggle to see who would be on top, David and Paul were fighting a much more insidious battle with homophobia that precluded emotional intimacy in their relationship. Each man, though not consciously aware of his avoidance of the feminine, was confusing a cultural stereotype of masculinity with a prohibition not to be tender or affectionate toward his partner. Both men equated their need to be held, to express a need for closeness and tenderness, with what Richard Isay (1989) refers to as "the sissy boy syndrome." A complicated dynamic not dissimilar to posttraumatic stress syndrome, the fear of being labeled a sissy often undermines intimate gay male relationships in adulthood.

Early internalized negative messages often get played out in male couples, particularly in a culture that rewards male independence and stoicism. The ensuing damage to a gay man's self-esteem is part of the reparative work that must occur for satisfying male partnerships to be created and must be addressed in a couple's treatment. Otherwise, male couples will often end treatment caught in circular patterns of behavior that appear to an observer as power struggles but are actually expressions of the gay men's struggles for acceptance and intimacy.

This reparative work is in addition to the structural maps or images created by the therapist during the enactment phase of treatment and is another way in which the treatment of male couples differs from the treatment of heterosexual couples. Although many individuals in heterosexual relationships have experienced traumatic ruptures in the development of their identity as a couple, these threats to the development of a consolidated identity are ubiquitous for gay people we see in our practices. If not addressed in family sessions, the internalized homophobia creates defensive behavioral patterns that interfere with the establishment of fulfilling relationships.

As the therapist watched and listened to Paul and David's common reactions to their week-earlier videotaped session, he realized that they were enacting their own version of the "Marlboro Man" image. Historically, men who express a need to be held or comforted are often thought of as either sissies or pathetic excuses for real men. This phenomenon, though not unique to gay men, becomes exacerbated for them as the experiences of gay identity formation and male acculturation interact. Allport (1958) wrote about the insidious nature of prejudice. According to Allport, the minority population either internalizes and acts out the stereotypes attributed to them or emulates an exaggerated image of the majority culture. The therapist reflected that David and Paul appeared to be reenacting outdated cultural stereotypes that "real men" are not affectionate, conciliatory, or dependent.

Often, to underscore the insights of an enactment for a couple, the therapist will register surprise even though he had anticipated the couple's interaction. However, in Paul and David's case, the therapist was genuinely saddened to hear how carefully they had constructed a relationship based on a stereotyped male image. Their dilemma reverberated within the session as all three men recognized the internalization of this ideal male, bereft and disconnected from the gay self. The therapist nodded in agreement as he identified with their experiences. Both the therapist and the couple were tearful as they acknowledged the destructiveness that homophobia can wreak among intimate male relationships.

The therapist encouraged Paul and David to talk to each other about their early experiences of knowing that they were gay. Each had been shamed for his gayness—Paul had painful memories of being mocked by other boys for his lack of athletic ability and David for his desire to play house with the girls. Both men made a connection at a young age that these shaming experiences happened because other children knew they were queer. During adolescence, neither dated and each carefully constructed a life that protected his gay identity from others. Paul joined the debate team and excelled, while David submerged himself in theater activities. Neither dated a man before college or graduate school. Paul talked about his first clandestine sexual experiences with men having taken place in porn shops and in public parks.

This was David's first long-term relationship and Paul's second. Both men were anxious and fearful as they experimented with compromise and negotiated their needs for affection with another man. David feared that once again he would get his childhood label of sissy for expressing his desire to be a homemaker. Paul was anxious that he would lose his manhood if he allowed David to lead him.

At this stage of the treatment, the couple's new insight into their enactments led naturally to the exploration of new behaviors. The couple's arguments began to diminish once they began to label these cultural chains for what they were. As the therapist encouraged the couple to experiment with new, softer behaviors toward each other, he labeled the construction of their relationship "The Dance of the Two Bulls," a phrase that acknowledged both their masculinity and their desire to be close to each other.

REVIEW OF ENACTMENTS

Each of the four couples presented in this chapter initially had some version of a linear explanation for their relational difficulties: Luke's challenging behavior made Fred anxious, Don's drug use threatened Gerry, Ernie wanted to open up his relationship with James, and Paul wished to end his relationship with David. The therapeutic use of enactments revealed the interpersonal dynamics that each couple had constructed. As opposed to a couple telling a therapist about the dynamics of their relationship, these in-session experiences of each couple's reality gave the therapists the information each needed to expand the definition of the couple's problems. Initially each partner blamed the other for his unhappiness. Through the enactments, the couples and the therapists experienced how each couple mutually maintained their circular patterns of behavior.

An additional level of treatment is necessary in working with male couples; family therapists need to be aware of the interactive effects of gender acculturation and the traumatic effects the men had experienced during gay identity formation. These shame-based experiences challenged the men's ability to form intimate relationships. In the case of David and Paul, the therapist had made a critical clinical error when he failed to pay sufficient attention to the men's stages of gay identity formation, in attempting to understand whether each had been able to consolidate his identity. The anxiety each man experienced from the foreclosure of his gay identity, expressed as a revulsion of same-sex affectionate expression, was being turned on the other partner. Couple treatment is the ideal context for reparative experiences when one or both individuals have foreclosed on the formation of his gay identity.

The case of Ernie and James demonstrated how gay couples are at risk due to marginalization by the majority culture. Bereft of role models, Ernie's preferred emotional style was disengagement—expressed through his desire to open their relationship. Whether in a "fight or flight" response that circumvents conflict, an avoidance of dependency needs, or a fear of being labeled a sissy, many gay men are conditioned to defend against their needs for softness and affection with a male partner. The next phase of treatment, unbalancing, will provide the systemic therapist with some case examples of how we provide gay couples with opportunities to engage in new, more complex, behaviors.

CHAPTER SIX

Unbalancing

Discovering New Steps

A NEW DANCE

Once a therapist has observed several interactions, or enactments, between a couple, the presenting problem can be reframed and expanded. From a linear explanation, where one partner generally blames the other, the therapist expands the presenting problem to include the couple's mutual complementary behaviors that maintain the symptom. In the case presented of Don and Gerry, the therapist expanded the meaning of the symptom—Don's recreational drug use while attending circuit parties—so that it became an interpersonal issue between the two men. The therapist reframed Gerry's presentation of the couple's problem as he observed their enactment: Don is lonely and wants to get Gerry's attention. Gerry appears focused on his prior relationship with his wife and son, ignoring his partner's concerns. During sessions Don expresses his loneliness as anger, having the paradoxical effect of pushing Gerry away.

In another case, Paul and David's circular patterns were also reframed. Paul and David presented with the classic symptoms of a couple who had outgrown their complementary relationship of protégé–mentor. Initially caught up in the content of their interactions, the therapist inadvertently discovered, through the playback of the videotaped enactments, the homophobia that was at the root of the men's inability to be affectionate with each other.

138

Enactments are generally a challenge for a therapist. Couples, although committed to homeostasis and fearful of change, are generally relieved once a therapist is able to reframe their problem from an individual to a systemic construction. Enactments, though, initially instill fear in a new family therapist, as the therapist must become directive with the couple, risking creating a situation of emotional intensity and the potential for the session to get out of the therapist's control.

Conversely, the unbalancing phase of the model often creates panic in the hearts of the couple as they experience ambivalence about giving up their preferred style of relating to explore new interactions. The task for the therapist during the unbalancing phase of treatment is relatively simple: hold up a mirror in which the couple may observe their own dance, to encourage them to experiment with new steps, new ways of interacting.

Unbalancing is a two-step process that directly follows a couple's enactments. First, using the language of complementarity, the therapist reflects what he has just observed in the enactment. "Don, when you take out a baseball bat and go after Gerry, you knock him out." "Gerry, when you closed down just now, it looked to me like Don gets lonelier and withdraws." Then, the therapist introduces novelty. "Gerry, see if you can reassure Don that you're his partner now." "Don, see if you can try some new behavior that will draw Gerry closer to you." The therapist's job is relatively easy at this stage of treatment. He reflects what he saw the couple do to each other and then he introduces novelty to the system as he invites the couple to experiment with new behavior.

Challenging couples to try a new dance, creating an environ that supports couples to experiment with new ways of being, presumes that the therapist believes that relationships can change. Inherent in the philosophy of the model are several beliefs: individuals are motivated toward healthy relationships; interdependency and responsibility toward others are healthy states of being; and we inherently have strengths that are underutilized in our connectedness with significant others. The therapist, observing a couple's interactions during their enactments, uses herself as the agent of change. She challenges the couple to become more resourceful and creative, unbalancing their status quo. The case of Truman and Donald will help to illustrate the unbalancing stage of the model.

MAKING A NEW HOME

Truman and Donald had been together for 8 years when they called for an appointment. They were wondering if they should end their relationship. They had met during graduate school and had lived together in Boston after graduation and before moving to New York a year ago. Both men grew up in northern New England, and each came from a conservative WASP family supportive of their coupled relationship. A year after they had moved in together, they had a commitment ceremony. Both families participated in the ceremony, and several generations— from grandparents to nieces and nephews—gathered to celebrate their union.

As the therapist joined with them in their first session, he was impressed with the strength of their relationship and the ease of their personal styles. With the exception of an emotional flatness in their relationship, they appeared to be a model couple.

The therapist was perplexed as to why they were in his office and asked, "Why are you here? You both appear so contented." Each of the men looked sad. Truman almost inaudibly said, "Donald doesn't want to sleep with me anymore." Over the past year, since moving to New York, Truman said they had stopped sleeping together. Truman had been offered a high-powered job as a financial analyst in New York and, for the first time in his career, was working 12-hour days. Donald had changed his own career to accommodate Truman's desire to take the new job.

Early on during the sessions, Donald had been silent but now the therapist wanted to hear his version of their problem. He asked Donald what the move had been like for him. Although Donald said he enjoyed his new career in sales, "I miss our home and friends," he admitted. Further exploration revealed that, since moving to New York, the couple had not replaced the network of friends that they had left behind in the Boston suburbs. As they talked about their new home, the therapist observed, "It sounds as if you are camping out and have never gotten unpacked." Truman nodded in agreement. He talked about having little free time and said that he often worked evenings and occasionally even went into the office on weekends.

Gradually the couple began to reveal the more threatening aspects of their presenting problem. Several months ago, Donald had begun to go outside the relationship, initially through contact on the Internet, for sexual encounters with other men. Truman, initially shocked by the discovery, eventually challenged Donald. They had talked briefly about this and agreed that henceforth each could have sexual encounters with other men, so long as there was no emotional involvement. Although intellectually open to the concept, Truman had found the arrangement difficult in practice. In becoming sexual with another man, Truman discovered that he inevitably became emotionally involved, and, this violated their basic agreement in opening up their relationship. Furthermore, Truman said matter-of-factly that he resented the secretiveness of Donald's liaisons and his continued disinterest in Truman's sexual advances. The therapist asked the two men to discuss this arrangement as they seemed to have different needs—or at least Truman did—that were not being met in their new arrangement.

We generally take a neutral stance on whether a couple should have an open or closed relationship. Monogamous relationships serve many purposes for heterosexual couples. Besides meeting emotional needs and providing stability for some people, monogamy is intended to preserve the bloodlines of progeny to ensure that estate and inheritance rights are maintained. For a minority of gay couples who are emotionally nurtured by their relationship and where they have both agreed, open relationships may work. However, we should state that in our combined clinical experience, we have worked with only a few couples who have successfully negotiated the permeability of boundaries that an open relationship requires so that neither partner feels threatened by the other's sexual encounters. Perhaps there is something in our emotional makeup as human beings that yearns for exclusivity in an intimate relationship. Additionally, in contemporary society there is the reality that most couples have two careers. Two-career families only have a limited amount of time and energy to be together. One partner can feel resentful if the other is out with someone else when they could be together. There is also the danger of sexually transmitted diseases being introduced into the relationship when the boundaries are open.

Politically the choice to open a relationship can be attractive because it makes a statement. For many gay couples an open relationship expresses their rejection of the majority's cultural norms, which gay people have often experienced as repressive. Some couples have told us emphatically, "But we don't want to be like the heterosexuals!" Refusing to be sexually monogamous may represent one of several ways that gay men insist on being autonomous. However, it takes a stable couple with high levels of self-esteem who are willing to negotiate with each other frequently to make open relationships work successfully. Open relationships that are successful are the exception rather than the norm.

In the case of Truman and Donald, the therapist set up an enactment, asking the two men to discuss with each other how this new arrangement was working for them. What became apparent to the therapist during this enactment was the depressed affect that characterized the men's interactions. Truman was the more verbal of the two. He talked to Donald in measured intellectual tones as he expressed his resentment that he had made an agreement not to date or get emotionally involved with anyone else. Donald did not make eye contact with him. Truman said, "I feel ashamed since I contracted hepatitis in going outside our relationship." Although he had not infected Donald, he said he was frightened by the experience. He wanted to be sexually intimate with Donald, but he no longer felt comfortable initiating intimacy.

Significant in this interaction was Donald's lack of any response. As the enactment had been set up, Donald was instructed to move off the sofa and to sit in a chair opposite from his partner. As Truman went on in a monologue, Donald sat in his chair with his head bowed, saying nothing. The therapist asked Donald if this was how he related to Truman at home, feeling quite certain that the absence of intensity observed in the enactment was symptomatic of the depressed character of their relationship. Donald nodded and said, "Yes." (It's interesting to note here how the therapist chose not to focus on the content of the couple's enactment so much as the nonverbal aspects of their interactions, e.g., their depressive affect and Donald's bowed head.)

Donald remarked that Truman tended to be the more verbal of the two and they generally avoided any conflict. The therapist said, "That's interesting because in my experience couples who can't disagree often have trouble making love. I don't know if you can have one without the other." Truman and Donald looked sorrowfully at the therapist. The therapist appeared to resonate with their conflict-avoidant style as he then spent the rest of the session and the next engaged in listening to their family histories as he did a genogram of each man's family. Not surprisingly, each of the men reported he had come from a family that disparaged emotional conflict.

It's unusual for a structural family therapist to do a genogram during this early stage of treatment. As the therapist joins with a couple, the initial focus is on identifying the interactional patterns of the system, exploring with the partners how they have mutually constructed their roles together. Structural therapists avoid genograms at this early stage of treatment because generally they diffuse the focus of treatment and lower the intensity of the couple's "here and now" experience of the session. Genograms move the couple to privilege cognitive strengths as they describe familial patterns of behavior. Generally, it is not until the middle stages of treatment, and then only if a therapist becomes stuck in unbalancing a couple's dance, that we will take a three-generation linear history of each partner's family. If the therapist decides to do a genogram, the goal is for each partner to discover how he was prepared for the role he has created in his current relationship and how he came to value the narrow way with which he now relates to the other. A therapist then has information that may help a couple expand their limited ways of relating to each other.

As the therapist did the genogram, both men revealed they were in recovery from alcohol addiction. Donald reported that he came from a family where there had been several generations of alcoholism. When conflict erupted in his family, Donald disconnected and learned to be self-sufficient as a child. Truman, on the other hand, came from a family where he had been a peacemaker between his mother and father. Although he had predictably failed at this impossible role for a child, he learned to be a soother to help his mother with her despondency over the loss of her husband. As is true for most couples, they had replicated a version of these roles in their adult relationship with one another. Truman had been an emotional soother to his mother, and he had sought out a partner whom he could soothe. Donald had found in Truman a partner who also valued low conflict. Putting peace and emotional safety on such a pedestal had created a relationship where neither man could express deeper needs, for fear of upsetting the status quo.

As this was their first session, the therapist felt it was important to leave Truman and Donald with a feeling of hope for their relationship. This strategy is useful for all couples but particularly important when working with gay couples, who are often isolated from sources of support. The therapist said: "Our time is up for today. How wonderful that in this world you found one another...someone who shares similar values of not expressing harsh feelings. However, this style of relating may not be helpful right now, 8 years into your relationship. You know, couples need to reinvent themselves every 7 or 8 years, and I wonder if you aren't struggling to do just that."

THE THERAPIST STRUGGLES TO AVOID BEING ORGANIZED BY SESSION CONTENT

The content of this couple's story was seductive and common as a presenting problem. Donald was having an affair with the Internet and all its romantic possibilities. As Truman brought in the symptom bearer, it was the therapist's unspoken job to fix Donald. The process level of this couple's lives told a more complex story. During the subsequent week, the therapist thought about this couple and where they appeared to be stuck. The relationship felt dead to the therapist; it was devoid of energy. Neither man had much affect. They were overly polite in session. Although they had been a couple for many years, they were without supportive resources since their move and appeared to have come to treatment for the therapist to fix their relationship. The therapist knew he needed to bring some life into the session. He felt like he had joined too well with them, and had easily adopted the couple's unemotional behavioral pattern.

The therapist decided to step up the intensity level during the next session to see if he could unbalance the partners preferred style of conflict avoidance. His hypothesis was that the flatness that he experienced in session with them was similar to an individual's depression. In this instance the couple's system was depressed. Like depression in an individual, which can be anger turned inward on the self, couples can become depressed when anger has no outlet. For Donald and Truman to express their anger might be therapeutic, as more open conflict might lead them to make positive changes in their system.

At the next session, the couple showed up early and appeared to be eager to begin. However, once the session began, they sat quietly, Donald looking at the floor and Truman looking at the therapist as if to say, "What should we talk about?" The therapist asked them if they had any thoughts about the first session. Neither said anything. The silence was deafening.

The therapist then asked how the week had gone for the two of them. Again, they offered a perfunctory "Fine," and the silence continued.

A therapist's use of self is important at moments like this. He is a "weather vane," testing the emotional wind patterns. This therapist felt quite ineffectual. He knew the couple was doing something to him that was akin to how they had constructed their relationship. The therapist needed to raise the intensity in the session, but he continued to feel inducted into their emotional style of low intensity. Perhaps anxious himself for fear of the conflict that might erupt if he continued to wait for one of the men to take responsibility for the session, he decided to take a history of their day-to-day routine. He rationalized to himself that he might not yet be sufficiently joined with the couple, and he requested of them: "Tell me what a typical day is like for you as a couple, from the moment you get up until the time you go to bed." This mode of inquiry can be helpful during the early joining stages as it is not confrontational and it provides the therapist with a great deal of information about how much time the couple spend together, whether they have a division of labor, and how well they accommodate each other's needs. However, this line of inquiry generally does not elicit much affect, as the therapist remains central in the session.

Truman spoke about the intensity of his weekday work schedule, getting up while it was still dark to take a commuter train that didn't return him home until 8 o'clock each evening. He then would have some dinner and be in bed by 9 or 9:30, only to begin the routine all over again the following day. Weekends were spent catching up on sleep or doing chores he couldn't find time to do during the week. Although he liked his new position as a financial analyst, his life sounded to the therapist like pure drudgery. All work and no time for one's partner can spell the death of a relationship.

Donald, on the other hand, reported a much less intense work life. He had begun a new career in sales since they had moved to the metropolitan area, and, although he often went to work for a few hours on Saturday, he generally was home by 5 or 6 in the evening. When the therapist asked what he did with his spare time, he said, "Nothing." He reported eating dinner alone in front of the television. Truman would join him for an hour or so when he got home, and they would watch TV together as Truman ate leftovers. When Truman went to bed, Donald would stay up watching the late news and often fell asleep on the sofa.

The therapist asked how this routine differed from the one they had when they lived on Boston's North Shore. Both men came alive as they spoke of the life they had left behind. They had lived in an old farmhouse that they had lovingly restored together. Truman was a gourmet cook and would often get out of work by 4:30, giving him enough time to shop and prepare a delicious dinner in the evening. Donald spoke with pride about the flower and vegetable garden that he had cultivated in their backyard. Suddenly, they seemed like a couple.

The therapist thought the aliveness that he experienced as they recalled memories of their former home might be an entrance into their dilemma, an opportunity to challenge their current state of disconnectedness. Donald no longer seemed to be the problem. The current absence of a "we-ness" in their relationship was the problem. Truman and Donald had lost each other in the process of relocating their common residence.

"Donald," the therapist said, "you came alive when you were talking about your life as a couple before coming to New York. Do you miss the Truman you married?"

He murmured a mournful "Yes."

The therapist, reframing their problem, then said, "Talk to him. Going outside the relationship may not be the only way of getting his attention. Talk to Truman about missing him."

Tentatively Donald began to talk about his loneliness. Initially he tried to talk to the therapist, and the therapist with the motion of his hand simply redirected him to address his comments to Truman. Donald was shy and uncomfortable talking directly to his partner. The therapist created the context for that interaction by physically moving him from his position beside Truman to a chair so that his back was partially to the therapist and he had to face Truman. With the therapist's support, Donald began to open up. Gradually, his voice went from being flat and void of affect, to expressing resentment for feeling abandoned. Donald, at first tentatively, expressed anger that their move to New York had been primarily for Truman's career advancement and at the expense of their relationship. He spoke about missing the gourmet dinners that Truman once made for them and the sense of "home" that eating together had created for him. Donald ended by saying he no longer felt they had a home together.

Truman sat silent. The therapist encouraged Truman to respond.

Although he hadn't been aware of Donald's feelings, Truman said he had consciously stopped preparing dinners as a way of expressing his resentment with Donald's extramarital excursions. "Your physical avoidance of me doesn't make me want to make a home with you."

As they got near the end of the second session, the therapist reinforced the good work that they were doing in opening up to each other about the feelings of loneliness that they were both experiencing in their disconnectedness. "You're expanding your style and the way you relate with each other. It's hard work, but you both appear to be much more energized."

The therapist then asked them if they would be willing to do something for each other during the next week, before the next session. They both seemed eager until the therapist made his request. He prefaced the request by saying that they needed to try something different, as they both seemed miserable and disconnected under the current arrangement. "Would you be willing to stop having outside sexual relationships for now? Let's say you close the relationship for the time that you are in treatment with me. Let's say 12 weeks?" Neither man jumped at this request. Donald said he was hesitant because he thought that closing the relationship would be a signal to Truman that he was ready to be intimate with him. He didn't have that desire. Truman seemed less reticent but wasn't hopeful that this agreement would be effective. Despite their reservations, they both agreed to close the relationship to outside sexual partners. "Truman," the therapist said, "since this seems to be something that Donald is doing for you, what would you be willing to do for him this week?" He thought for a few seconds and said that he would prepare a home-cooked gourmet meal over the weekend. Donald seemed pleased, and the session ended.

During the following week, the therapist thought about what he had asked the couple to do. It seemed they had been putting very little energy into their relationship. Like many professional couples, one or both of them gave everything at the office and neither had anything left to bring home. The therapist was asking them to reconsider their priorities and focus more energy into their relationship. In making a homework assignment, the therapist had no way of knowing whether the couple would sabotage the assignment or what, if any, effect the request to observe monogamy would have on the relationship. However, the couple's style of relating had definitely changed during the session. Donald's voice had become much clearer as he expressed his anger over Truman's putting his work above their relationship. It's interesting to observe systemically how the couple's gripes about the deadness in their relationship had diminished as Donald's anger and sadness at feeling abandoned by Truman surfaced.

REFRAMING THE PROBLEM: CIRCULAR CAUSALITY

The therapist had no way of predicting this expansion of the couple's presenting problem, as he initially was unable to make a structural map.

He was aware that he didn't hear Donald's voice in the sessions and that the relationship felt depressed. His objective in the session had been to raise the couple's affect level so that the feelings they were repressing might find a voice. What happened, and how, became clearer as Donald and Truman disclosed the details of their lives as a couple before, and after, their move to New York. The therapist began to think of Donald's extramarital liaisons as an indirect way of expressing his loneliness and his anger. Donald's behavior led the therapist to make a connection to Truman's long hours away from their home. It was a reframe that the therapist created; he had no way of knowing if it would resonate with the couple.

For therapists new to structural work, the use of reframes can often appear counterintuitive. This couple's presenting problem was that they were considering breaking up. Truman then revealed his dissatisfaction with Donald for his being sexually and emotionally unavailable. Donald appeared silent and withdrawn. If the therapist was thinking linearly and caught in content, Donald would have been the patient. He held the symptoms for this system. However, for the therapist to accept the couple's story would have been simplistic. The couple's explanation of their dilemma was too one-dimensional.

To introduce novelty, we view families with multidimensional lenses that permit an expansion of the problem to make it a relational one. The art of family therapy is how to expand the problem from a linear one—"Fix Donald and our relationship might be salvageable"—to a circular one that says the couple are jointly responsible for creating a relationship that feels barren and bereft of nurturance. This concept of complementary behaviors that result in predictable patterns of behavior for a couple (Bateson, 1979) guided the therapist in his creation of the reframe. Donald betrayed Truman when he went outside the relationship. He needed to take responsibility for that betrayal. Simultaneously, Truman must recognize his role in this dynamic. Truman asked Donald to move to a new city to accommodate his career advancement. He then buried himself in his new job, leaving Donald to fend for himself. Without excusing Donald's betrayal of Truman, the therapist expanded the problem by creating a reframe, namely, "Could you find another way to get Truman's attention?" The couple's problem was not simply that Donald has had outside sexual partners. Their relationship had lost its vitality as Truman focused on his career and they needed to re-infuse it with life.

An additional level of work that is frequently necessary when working with male couples is for the therapist to address the psychological dynamics that have occurred during the formation of each man's gay identity. Otherwise, structural interventions that unbalance a couple's preferred relational style temporarily may not lead to permanent change. In order for a couple to become closer, they must experiment with novel ways of relating to each other. The therapist creates a safe space for the men to experiment with new behaviors that expose their vulnerability, fear of rejection, and needs for dependency and affiliation. So, although we use the word "challenging" to indicate how we unbalance a couple in this phase of treatment, we are often giving a male couple permission to access the softer, more feminine side of themselves. A therapist may spend many sessions interrupting the old patterns of relating and then reinforcing the new interdependent behaviors during the unbalancing phase of treatment.

The next session, their fourth, the couple once again was early and again appeared eager to begin. This time, however, they maintained an energetic enthusiasm. The therapist asked them how their week had gone, and they both grinned as they simultaneously said, "We had an argument." Their verbal disagreement had been about how to fix up their house so that it was more of a home. They said they had been sleeping on a futon since moving to New York. Over the weekend they decided to go out and purchase a new bed. The argument had been over what style of bed they should purchase.

The therapist commented that they both seemed much more alive, and he wondered if anything else had happened during the intervening week. Truman then talked about making Sunday dinner, and Donald spoke about the warm feelings he had as he smelled the roast cooking in the oven. He then mentioned, almost under his breath, that they had made love. The therapist was surprised at this sudden turn of events. He wanted to reinforce these new behaviors, so he asked Donald to talk with Truman about what Truman had done that made him want to be intimate. "Just last week, Donald, you had expressed a lack of interest in being close to Truman. Please, tell Truman what he did that made you want to be closer to him again."

Donald told Truman that when he saw him preparing dinner for them, he once again experienced loving feelings for him. He knew Truman must want to save the relationship, as he hadn't cooked in the house since they had moved in. Donald was touched by Truman's effort to reestablish an important ritual in their lives. Truman said that he was encouraged by Donald's efforts to arrange for them to play tennis doubles over the weekend, something that they both loved to do but had not done since moving. Donald knew a colleague who had a membership at a tennis club, and he had surprised Truman with the invitation to play with her and her partner over the next weekend.

As they talked about their fighting, playing, and lovemaking, the therapist reflected how stressful it must have been for them to move. The men talked for the first time about the loss each had experienced when they had given up the home they both had cherished and moved to a big city where they knew no one. Like many couples, rather than focusing on the external stresses of loss that the move had entailed, they had disconnected from each other. The task for Truman and Donald was now to reconnect and to learn to meet each other's needs in their new world.

As the session ended, the therapist said, "I see you creatively working as a couple to manage the stress of your move. How wonderful, Truman, that you have the ability to make Donald feel loved in your new home. Donald, how respectful of you to confront Truman with what you miss in him rather than choosing to disconnect."

They would need the reinforcement of several more sessions to solidify their new ways of being together. During that time, a crisis occurred when each of the men reverted back to their old behaviors. Truman discovered that Donald had gone back on the Internet chat lines. Truman was angry and went out for a beer. This occurred just after Truman had taken on a new project at his firm that required more of his time. Rather than talk about this additional stress, the men had relapsed into their avoidance mode of relating. However, once in session they identified their old pattern of behavior (i.e., when Truman distanced, Donald responded by also distancing). This time, they were able to reconnect more readily.

AN INVITATION TO PUT DOWN THE BAT: DON AND GERRY REVISITED

Generally speaking, enactments occur early in treatment and provide a therapist with the information needed to usefully reframe a couple's relational dynamic. The unbalancing of a couple's preferred style of relating can usually occur in three to six therapy sessions. During the remaining sessions, a therapist and a couple must use the time to reinforce new patterns of interacting. The duration of treatment depends upon how rigidified a couple are in their old behavior patterns and how motivated they are to change the dynamics of their relationship.

As the therapist takes a position that permits her to observe a couple's dynamics during the enactment phase of treatment, she simultaneously may identify possible interventions to unbalance a couple's preferred style of relating. The enactment is the play, to use the metaphor of theater, in which a therapist becomes the audience in order to observe the complementary roles of the players. Unbalancing is a challenge for the players to become the playwrights to rewrite their script.

Let's revisit the couple Don and Gerry, who had met while Gerry was still married, to see how they rewrote their script. Although Gerry's involvement with his son after he separated from his wife was beneficial to both the son and his son's mother, his continued social and financial arrangements with his former wife left Don feeling like "a third wheel." Gerry was bewildered as to how his actions might be contributing to Don's defiant behavior, and Don was equally unaware of how his behavior was driving Gerry toward his wife for companionship. Gerry's response to Don's rebellious behavior was to become parental with Don and speak to him as if he too was an adolescent son. "You're behaving irresponsibly. You could become addicted to drugs or contract a sexually transmitted disease. I don't understand why you're behaving this way."

The therapist intervened on Gerry's concrete concerns as he risked getting caught in the role of the couple's problem solver and Don's policeman. Gerry's concerns were legitimate and Don knew that. However, Don was not chemically dependent, and ultimately they were not coming to couple therapy to get a lecture on safer sex or the dangers of using Ecstasy.

After the therapist extricated himself from the role of cop, he could have taken one of many paths at this juncture in treatment. He knew that he needed to do something once he observed the enactment of the "father chastising the rebellious son." The simplest intervention, and one that might begin to challenge their father–son dynamic, would be for the therapist to hold up a mirror for them to observe what he had just seen. However, the therapist made a decision that might seem counterintuitive. At this early stage in treatment, he decided to introduce novelty as he challenged the couple's construction of their relationship by supporting Don.

The therapist thought that Don appeared by his rebellious behavior to be expressing his feelings of disempowerment in this system. The therapist felt that Don, unfortunately, was acting out his feelings of loneliness instead of (more constructively) confronting Gerry with what he was missing in their relationship. He said, "Don, can you tell Gerry what he does to you that makes you respond like a rebellious adolescent?" This was a two-pronged intervention, as it mirrored the dynamic that the therapist observed and challenged Don to be more proactive rather than reactive to Gerry's hierarchical position. Alternatively, the therapist could have reflected what he had observed by saying, "When you two talk with each other, it's as though a parent were speaking to a child." If he said nothing more, most likely the partners would have then turned to the therapist with some kind of comment, and once again the therapist would have become central to the session. If the goal is to keep the dynamic solely between the two men, the therapist needs next to add, "Don, talk to Gerry about how he makes you so rebellious."

It is for their emphasis on the unbalancing phase of treatment that structural family therapists take the most heat from postmodernists and the narrative school of therapy. Joining is common to all forms of therapy and elicits no criticism. Enactments are central to structural family therapy because of the focus on the couple relating in "the here and now" as opposed to reporting on their behavior outside of the treatment. Enactments in general are not provocative to postmodernists, since in enactments a therapist is simply asking a couple to speak to each other rather than to the therapist. However, the unbalancing phase of treatment is most controversial (Anderson & Goolishian, 1988). Challenging and unbalancing a couple's preferred style of interpersonal behavior is often labeled by postmodernists as "disrespectful," "bullying," "culturally insensitive," "hierarchical," and/or "patriarchal." We agree that all of these accusations can be true. Some therapists are guilty of imposing their own values, insensitively confronting families, and being ignorant of the cultural differences motivating others. Any therapeutic technique can be misused or abused, and all therapies share in common the injunction that a therapist always remain respectful of her clients. Respect for clients is a necessary condition that must be present in all treatments if there is to be a therapeutic alliance and any meaningful change in behavior.

But we believe that a therapist has expertise and leverage that can be used to benefit a couple. To deny that a therapist has advanced training and expertise in the dynamics of relational systems would be pointless. Choosing how to use the power of knowledge creatively requires the therapist to be both self-aware and ethical. The therapist intervenes based upon what is observed in the session. The therapist creates intensity by labeling and confronting the family's dynamic. The unbalancing phase of treatment is based upon a belief that people change their behavior when they reach a critical state of discomfort that becomes intolerable for both the individuals and the system. Members of the family at this stage have the opportunity to take responsibility for the consequences of their behavior.

The therapist's challenge to Don and Gerry's complementary behavior was to label their problem as disconnectedness rather than strictly Don's abuse of recreational drugs and partygoing. If the therapist had wanted to support Gerry more directly, he could have said to him, "Tell Don what he does that makes you talk to him like an adolescent." Or if he deliberately wanted to be less challenging with Don, he might have said, "Don, you seem to keep Gerry busy watching and worrying about you. Have you ever been successful in getting his attention?" Don would then have responded to the therapist, and the therapist would then direct him to talk with Gerry about his loneliness, desire for more attention, or whatever it was that was motivating his behavior. What is essential and central to structural family therapy is for a therapist to turn the dynamic back to a couple for them to negotiate new roles and ways of relating to each other. The therapist's role is to use his observational skills to be a facilitator of change.

We take an intermediate or back seat during this stage of treatment, when the couple is encouraged to invent a new dance. If the therapist is adequately joined with and respectful of a couple, she may nonetheless err with interventions that have too little or too much intensity. The therapist, listening to her own emotional responses to the couple, uses her feelings as a barometer to gauge whether her interventions have created sufficient intensity for the couple to engage in new behaviors. Videotaped recordings of the sessions, as well as live supervision, can also help a therapist to monitor the effectiveness of her interventions.

Initially, the therapist's attempts to reframe the problem and to un-balance Don and Gerry were not effective. They did not have the effect of making Don's behavior dystonic for him. Rather than try new ways to engage Gerry, Don responded with greater obstinancy, sometimes di-recting Gerry's attention to their own father–son dynamic. He increas-ingly got incensed and said he deserved to be out with his friends. He reiterated that he had stayed home like a dutiful partner for many years or vacationed with Gerry's former wife and son, and he now intended to enjoy himself. Don's anger was impressive and appeared to paralyze Gerry. However, his anger was not having the potentially desirable effect of changing Gerry's behavior. To be an effective agent of change, the therapist knew that his next intervention needed to uncover some of the abandonment and hurt that Don's angry behavior was masking. Otherwise, Don's anger would not promote growth in their relationship. The therapist switched his focus to Gerry. "Gerry, do you know when it was that Don decided he was single and started to go to circuit parties? Were you ever able to make him feel like he was your partner?"

Gerry responded that he thought he did make Don feel special early on in their relationship. After he moved into Don's apartment a couple of years ago, though, something had happened where he felt Don became more distant. "He always seemed to be angry at me," Gerry said. There were several ways that the therapist could intervene at this point. Gerry's use of the phrase "Don's apartment" was an indication that they may have never successfully created a couple's identity as a separate entity. This hypothesis was strengthened by the information that the two families (Don and Gerry, and Gerry's son and his mother) continued to share a vacation home and often spent vacation time to-gether.

The therapist chose to stay with the current interaction and in-crease the intensity. "Gerry, have you ever found out why Don's so angry at you?" He replied, quite innocently, "No." The therapist said the obvi-ous, "He's here, why don't you ask him."

Couples, like individuals in treatment, teach a therapist in many different ways what they need to know about them. There is no one right way—nor is there only one path—to help a couple to relate with each other in new ways. Although Don continued to be defensive, he cautiously began to talk with Gerry about the resentment he had built up. Don told Gerry that, by refusing to divorce his former wife, Gerry made him feel as though he was involved in an illicit relationship. The fact that Gerry continued to own property jointly with his wife made Don question Gerry's commitment to their common future as a family. To his credit, Gerry was able to hear Don's pain beneath the anger. It was obvious to the therapist that Gerry wanted to strengthen his relationship with Don.

Gerry began to make changes in his life that moved him closer to Don. Over the next couple of weeks, Gerry met with his wife. As a result, they put their jointly owned real estate on the market and drew up a divorce settlement. Gerry's willingness to hear Don's concerns and his responding with new behavior that communicated his commitment and concern for his partner gave Don the courage to begin to examine his own behavior. He began to listen to Gerry's concerns for his well-being and asked Gerry for his help in discontinuing what he now recognized was destructive behavior.

Although Gerry and Don had been together for several years, like many gay couples who present for treatment, they were stuck in the early stages of creating an identity as a family. In this instance, though separated from his wife, Gerry had not completely disengaged from his first marriage. Perhaps a result of coparenting with his former wife, Gerry had not emotionally separated from her nor shifted his loyalties to his new partner, Don. This arrangement had worked well for the first few years of Don and Gerry's relationship as Don was focused on building a career. Eventually, though, as the two men entered middle age and their careers became less of a focus, Don became resentful of the amount of time that his partner spent with his former wife.

The need to establish an identity that says that a couple is a family with boundaries separate from other families is a task that all couples must negotiate. It is particularly challenging for new couples when one partner has children from a former marriage and must maintain a relationship with the former spouse for parental collaboration. The task for blended families is for the new couple to create an identity and for the parent to still stay in a parental role for the children. The task is complicated by two phenomena: the nonbiological spouse instantly inherits a family, and the spouse/parent needs to disengage emotionally and socially from the former spouse while maintaining his coparenting obligations. Additionally, gay couples must deal with the homophobia of their children, often particularly salient among adolescent boys, and the pressure they can feel to be "perfect parents" in a culture that often questions their right to parent at all (Martin, 1993).

What happened to Don and Gerry's relationship as they struggled with these tasks is more characteristic of gay male than heterosexual couples. Rather than Don's challenging his partner, saying that he felt lonely and abandoned in the relationship, Don disconnected from Gerry. Gerry, in response to Don's withdrawal, turned to his former wife for emotional nurturance. This is a dynamic—often referred to as the "Marlboro man syndrome" or its obverse form, the "sissy boy syndrome"—that we often see with men in general and even more frequently with gay men. What we don't see, however, is the extraordinary price that men pay, usually through deterioration of their health, either in the avoidance of or, in the latter case, the fulfillment of this cultural fantasy.

Don had responded to the insecurity he felt with Gerry in fairly predictable ways. He became angry, suppressing his needs for closeness, and he became detached. Treatment created the space where both men's needs for intimacy with each other could be normalized and expressed. Once the therapist had sufficiently joined with the couple and he had identified the couple's difficulty in creating an identity as the real problem, the therapy began to focus on supporting Don's voice so that he could be more open with Gerry about his feelings of loneliness. Subsequently the therapist helped the couple to become clearer on what tasks Gerry needed to do to continue to coparent adequately but also to separate from his former wife. Gerry got the courage to do this when he realized that Don would not abandon him and was committed to the longevity of their relationship. The couple was fortunate in that they did not have to contend with any lack of acceptance from either the son or his mother.

As we mentioned earlier, there is not the same taboo against extramarital relationships for gay couples as exists for heterosexual couples. However, as treatment progressed with Don and Gerry, what initially looked like mutually agreeable open arrangement became more clearly a weapon that Don used to express his anger and sadness over Gerry's emotional absence in their relationship. Don initially had difficulty expressing his vulnerability to Gerry. He acted out his feelings of hurt by expressing either anger or disconnecting from the relationship. Don was ashamed to admit that he needed Gerry to be more present in his life. Not only did he believe it "unmanly" to express such dependent feelings, but when Don felt himself to be in need of Gerry, he reexperienced the traumatic feelings of being labeled a queer when he was an adolescent in high school. In one emotional session he told Gerry how he had become very aware of his atypical behavior as a teenaged boy as he realized that he was gay and attracted to boys and not girls. The boys on the football team taunted him for not being athletic and called him a "duck" (a euphemism for "faggot") due to the way he walked. He told Gerry that early in his development, he had made a decision never to show his vulnerable side to anyone, especially not to a man who could potentially ridicule him for being different.

Gerry, in contrast, had grown up oblivious to the type of early childhood trauma that Don had suffered. Gerry had grown up dating girls and felt very much accepted by the majority culture and his peers. In high school he had been an athlete and participated in many extracurricular activities. Repressing his attraction to men, he had dated girls through college and had been very popular, taking up a leadership position in his university government. His formative years were a world apart from the trauma that Don had experienced as he hid an essential aspect of who he was.

Though Don had endured significant childhood trauma, he was further along as an adult in integrating his gay identity than Gerry. Don was out to his immediate and extended family and had been so since college. Initially uncomfortable in expressing his desire for closeness with Gerry, once he experienced the therapist's support, Don found his voice. Though unaccustomed to feeling safe in expressing tenderness and his desire to be held by Gerry, Don needed little coaching by the therapist to access that side of himself. He teared up as he expressed his desire to be held by Gerry.

Gerry, not having come out until he was well into his 20s, was initially overwhelmed to hear Don's intimate language. Gerry also was desirous of exploring his sexual attraction for other men, feeling that he had missed out on this aspect of his life during his early adulthood. Don began to teach Gerry how to be more comfortable talking about his own needs for emotional closeness. The men became physically more comfortable with each other as they expressed affection that no longer needed to be exclusively expressed through sexual encounters. Couple treatment provided both men with a safe and supportive environment for them to experiment with being more interdependent. As treatment ended, Gerry surprised Don with plans for a trip to Europe that included just the two of them.

Gay men often fear that disagreement will inevitably lead to physical blows and/or the repetition of shaming experiences. If a family therapist is willing to model vulnerable behavior and help a male couple explore their fears, he can normalize the needs for closeness that are an essential element in intimate relationships. In these situations couple therapy is a healing and corrective experience for gay men and can be an inspiration for the therapist. Gay men, once they realize that they are not going to be shamed for expressing needs for affection and support by another man, often become very creative in their relationships (Green et al., 1996). They often realize that they are free to let go of cultural stereotypes.

REVISITING THE CARETAKER AND HIS PATIENT

For a gay man to have a healthy self-image it may not always be necessary for him to come out to his family. In some cases, as Green et al. (1996) have observed, coming out may destabilize a relationship or be counterproductive for a gay man. However, in the case of Ernie and James, the issue was not coming out about their individual gay identities but rather coming out as a couple. Ernie and James were struggling with loyalty and affiliation issues related to Ernie's financial arrangements with his biological family. These issues of parity were highly similar to what Ernie and James had been working on as a couple in treatment.

As Ernie and James argued over how to allocate their funds for the month, the therapist could have chosen many ways to intervene. Discussions about combining or pooling of funds represented a new stage in their commitment to each other that had occurred only since they had been in couple treatment. Prior to the recent establishment of a joint bank account, like many gay couples regardless of how long they have been together, they had kept separate funds. This common dynamic in gay couples reflects not only gender acculturation that emphasizes male independence and control but also the lack of legalization of same-sex unions. The couple had decided only recently to try a new way of being together financially that reflected both Ernie's new job status and the couple's deepening commitment to each other. Now they needed to negotiate how they would allocate their resources. Ernie had not revealed to his parents that he used their stipend for the couple's household expenses. He feared his parents would withdraw their support if they discovered that he and James were a couple and had a joint bank account.

The therapist said, "You have a dilemma as a couple. Ernie's parents are telling you to remain single. What are you going to do?"

Their immediate response was not a solution, but it relieved the tension that the therapist's challenge had created. "We'll just lie to them," said Ernie. Both men laughed, and the session ended with the matter unresolved.

A week later, as the couple entered the therapist's office, each had a bemused look on his face. They sat beside each other and appeared to be joined in some conspiratorial plot. Almost gleefully Ernie said, "We have a surprise for you." He took out a letter that he had written to his parents and read it to the therapist.

Dear Mom and Dad,

James and I have decided to write to you and clarify some things which may not be apparent to you. We want to do this because you have been so generous financially and we don't think it's fair to accept your help if you don't understand what our relationship is. We are life partners. We want you to think of us as a married couple.

During our phone conversations, although you've never said this explicitly, I've gotten the impression that the money you send me is meant just for me and you don't want James to benefit from it. We understand this. I am your son and James is not. But it is not possible for you to help me exclusive of James.

Perhaps if I were straight and married to a woman you would think differently about this. You might not think twice about her and me sharing our finances. You might feel more comfortable about helping us establish a family in this economically challenging city and time. We want to encourage you to think of us as partners trying to establish a family. James works extremely hard and generates a large part of our income in his job. In addition, he is building a portfolio as a designer. He also is beginning to generate income from that, and our hope is that he will earn from that more and more frequently. When James gets a check from a freelance job, he does not keep it and say, "It's mine to spend however I want"—any more than either of you would withhold income from your relationship. He puts it toward our mutual financial responsibilities. When you help me financially, I do the same with that money.

We have been talking a lot about the issue of finances in our daily lives and couple therapy, and both of us in the coming year are hoping to increase our earning power and, as a result, decrease our dependence on you. We do rely on your help now, and are very grateful for it. But we feel it is unfair to you to accept it without clarifying our position. Unfair to you because it's your money and our situation may not be acceptable to you; unfair to us because it allows you to view me as a child and James as a friend rather than as two adults trying to establish a family. We hope we can continue to rely on your help, but, if this changes things for you, please let us know—and rest assured that your help thus far has been greatly appreciated.

Both men were delighted with the letter, and they appeared united as a couple for the first time since treatment had begun. James turned to Ernie and said, with great affection, how proud he was of him. He told Ernie that he had always wanted to be life partners with him but he had thought Ernie would never agree to that kind of commitment. Both men were concerned that Ernie's family might withdraw their financial stipend, but they seemed to take courage in the fact that they could pull together to make the relationship solvent. Although the couple had not found a magic cure for longevity, they were successfully negotiating the terrain of creating a boundary in their journey to be a family of their own. Like any couple, many obstacles lay ahead of them as they taught each other, day by day, to accommodate each other's needs.

REVIEW OF UNBALANCING

In the case examples presented in this chapter, the therapist unbalanced the couple's preferred style of interacting by challenging them to relate to each other in new ways. Fear of commitment, avoidance of conflict, and difficulties in creating an identity are challenges common to many couples. In the cases reviewed, in order for the therapist to successfully help the couples experiment with new behaviors the therapist had to attend to the interactional process of the session and not be inducted into solving the narrative problem that each couple presented with.

Truman and Donald were struggling with Donald's "cyber affairs" at the onset of treatment. After meeting with the couple, it was apparent to the therapist that the couple had difficulty in confronting each other with the needs that each had for greater intimacy. The couple was depressed, and the relationship was emotionally flat, a situation that had occurred after their move to a new city. As trust had to be reestablished in the relationship for the couple to rediscover each other, the therapist requested that they keep the relationship closed for the duration of treatment. The therapist's decision to ask them to do this was based on his assessment that the couple had lost intensity in their relationship by opening it up to multiple sexual partners, that is, they avoided conflict by redirecting sexual energy toward other men. The unbalancing and discovery of new ways of relating for the couple occurred as they began to negotiate with each other for more closeness—Donald's need for a greater sense of home and Truman's need for more physical closeness. Treatment provided the men with a safe place to begin to explore more ways to be vulnerable in their relationship. Each took risks in asking more of the other, and in the process their relationship became much more vital.

Don and Gerry presented for treatment with a very different set of problems. A couple for several years, they had successfully negotiated an open relationship. Gerry, however, was concerned about Don's recently defiant behavior, as he had begun to experiment with drugs at circuit parties. What the couple had never learned to talk about prior to treatment was Don's feelings of rejection. He had always felt like "a third wheel" in their relationship, since Gerry remained so loyal to his former wife and their son. Don didn't object to Gerry's parenting responsibilities and was fond of his partner's son. What he objected to was the sharing of their lives with Gerry's wife. Instead of taking "a baseball bat" as Don had to get Gerry's attention, the therapist reframed the problem as Don's needing to experiment with other ways to communicate his desire for closeness. Gerry simultaneously had to demonstrate to Don that he could acknowledge his partner's needs for closeness. This new openness created novelty for the couple as they made a deeper commitment to their relationship. Gerry turned less to his wife and more to Don for nurturance as he gained greater trust in their relationship. They continued to have an open relationship.

Similar to Don and Gerry, David and Paul, the hip downtown gay couple described in Chapter 5, were caught in a no-win dynamic when they entered treatment. The two men constantly argued over even the most trivial matters in their relationship. Having initially constructed a hierarchical relationship of mentor–protégé, once David had found his voice, they appeared to be caught in a seemingly unending symmetrical power struggle. As the therapist joined with the couple, they presented as being open and comfortable with their status as a gay couple. For a while the therapist got overinvolved in the content of the sessions, focusing on their power struggle, until by chance he discovered the homophobia that was repressing their natural inclinations to become a couple. Once the couple became aware of their fear of appearing effeminate or being stereotyped as "Chelsea boys," they were able to begin to negotiate their needs to take turns as the leader and the follower in their day-to-day life as a couple.

This avoidance of shameful homophobic labels that can hold all men, straight or gay, hostage to society's stereotypes can be extremely destructive for gay male couples. As family therapists, we must be aware of this dynamic even with the most liberated gay couples. If this society-wide dynamic is not addressed, the treatment will not produce long-term stability in a relationship. Family therapy sessions become a laboratory where gay men can experiment with new behaviors having to do with vulnerability, dependency, and softness. Male therapists especially need to be comfortable with their own feminine side and fully aware of any latent homophobia that might blind them to important aspects of a gay couple's struggles.

Ernie and James came into treatment having never created an identity as a couple—not unlike the dynamics that we see in many newly formed couples regardless of sexual orientation. Ernie's disclosure of his partnered relationship with James to his parents did not have the adverse reaction that the two men had feared. Ernie's parents did not withdraw their financial support, and they began to acknowledge the two men as a couple. Their coming out as a couple was an affirmation for the men. We cannot generalize this outcome. Ernie had been out to his parents and they accepted him as a gay *single* man. The issue for the couple was Ernie's need to differentiate from his own family. If his parents had not been accepting of his homosexuality or if they were from a culture that had no experience with same-sex couples, the therapist might not have supported the letter announcing their life partnership to Ernie's family. In working with gay couples, it is important for the therapist to realize that what works with one couple might be disastrous for another couple.

All the gay couples that presented benefited from being able to explore with each other how their own traumatic experiences as gay boys contributed to the creation of defenses that interfered with their intimate relationships as adults. Unlearning the culture's stereotypes for "what it means to be a man" is not an easy task; nor is deconstructing the presentation of the false self that results from such stereotypes. Often couples will return periodically for continued treatment. Gay couples need a safe place that honors their relationship and normalizes the struggles that they experience in creating a relationship that allows for dependency and softness.

The termination of treatment is normally a joint decision between the therapist and the couple. Generally speaking, after a few sessions in which the couple demonstrates new, more satisfying, behaviors, it's time for them to go out on their own and practice their new ways of being a couple. Gay couples, particularly ones that are isolated from support systems, may experience some anxiety during the termination process. As we do with most couples getting ready to terminate, the therapist can tell the couple not to feel defeated if they ever need to return for a few sessions. Paraphrasing Dr. Linda Carter, Director of Family Studies at the Child Study Center at NYU Medical Center, we tell our clients: "Families too can need a checkup—just as an individual goes to an internist for one."

CHAPTER SEVEN

A Case Study

Male Couples and Connectedness

This chapter is about the treatment of a gay male couple that has had a profound influence on the way we conceptualize the mission of couple therapy with gay men. Because the case so eloquently exemplifies the type of emotional connection men are capable of, we have transcribed several sessions of the therapy in detail. On the one hand, the progression of this 7-month treatment demonstrates the stages of the structural family model—joining, enactment, and unbalancing. But it is the last session that contains the seeds of what has become a primary focus in our work within the model: to help male couples create and maintain emotional connectedness. During their final session, only a few hours before one of the men died of AIDS, the couple demonstrated a depth of connectedness, compassion, and empathy that is seldom seen.

Coping with end-of-life issues can be excruciatingly painful for the individual, family, and loved ones. But clinical work at this time can also be extraordinarily rewarding. Families and couples often drop their defensive armor that in more normal times keeps them from listening to what the other needs and prevents them from responding supportively.

One of the authors met the couple for the first time 10 years ago during a clinical intake when he was director of family therapy training at an outpatient psychiatric clinic. Together 2 years, Seth and Jon presented initially with severe problems in communicating and were on the verge of breaking up. Both were HIV-positive when they met and had been symptom-free until a few months before the intake, when Seth had

164

developed his first opportunistic infection and was formally diagnosed with AIDS.

Seth, 40, had been a successful artist until becoming disabled by AIDS. Of short stature and with straight blond hair, he was boyish-looking but conveyed an attitude of quiet reserve and introspection. He had been raised in the South as an only child, and his father had died some years ago, leaving his mother as his only living relative. She lived 2 hours away in Philadelphia and visited frequently, more so since Seth had become ill. Seth had lost his previous partner to AIDS.

Jon, 36, was employed as an elementary teacher in a private school. Also HIV-positive, he showed no signs of illness. A quintessential and native New Yorker, Jon had grown up in the Bronx, the youngest of four children, with three older sisters. Jon, with his curly black hair and dark features, was lively and extremely outgoing, never at a loss for words. His mother had died of cancer when he was 8, with his oldest sister and his grandmother helping to raise him and the other siblings. Jon's father had died a few years ago, but Jon was never close to him. Jon was extremely close to a sister who lived nearby.

At the end of the intake, the author told the men he was assigning them to work with a psychology intern whom he knew had a specialty interest in working with families coping with serious illness.[1] He explained to them that, as part of being treated in a training clinic, most of their therapy sessions would be observed by him and other interns from behind a one-way mirror. This "team behind the mirror" would call in with their thoughts from time to time, and all sessions would be videotaped. The men gave their permission to be observed and videotaped, but immediately they voiced concerns about working with a woman whom they presumed to be straight.

"What does she know about gay men? What will she think about working with a male couple?" they asked. The supervisor suggested they meet the therapist and bring up their issues directly with her. They agreed to a first session. As they were leaving, Jon said we should know that he had been in individual therapy for many years. Perhaps anticipating where the therapy might be headed, Jon added, "I have unresolved issues with abandonment because, as I already told you, my mother died when I was 8."

---

[1] The psychology intern was Elena Taurke Joseph.

JOINING

In late September 1992 Jon and Seth met their therapist for the first time. By the end of the first meeting, the therapist managed to allay their concerns about whether she could understand a gay couple and had begun to forge a strong working relationship with them. She did this partly through her engaging and respectful style and partly by asking specific questions that left no doubt that she understood their lifestyle and respected them as a gay male couple. For example, she asked straightforwardly whether they were monogamous (they were). Later, when they told her they had been together 2 years, she asked, "Well, what date do you celebrate as your anniversary, and why did you choose that date?"

Like most male couples, Jon and Seth had an interesting story to tell in response to that question. And, as with many gay couples, these men celebrated the day they first met as their anniversary. The minute they laid eyes on each other, there had been an instant attraction that was more than sexual chemistry. Jon had been leaving his individual therapist's office one afternoon and was briefly sitting on the therapist's stoop crying quietly before getting on his bike. Seth happened to be walking by and smiled shyly at him. Always ready for an interaction, Jon responded to Seth's smile and struck up a conversation that continued through dinner and well into the night. By dawn the next morning, each felt a strong physical and emotional attraction to the other. After a year of dating, Seth moved in with Jon. They said they had dealt with HIV issues from the very beginning. As Jon said later, during the therapy, "With both of us being HIV-positive, we always knew that our relationship would end by one of us dying."

Fifteen minutes into the first session, after the requisite polite small talk, the therapist asked what specifically had brought the couple into therapy. Seth explained the situation as he perceived it:

> "I see a lot of different levels in which our lives are just going to be inexplicably interwoven . . . from the emotional to the physical . . . and I also see . . . big gaps where we are never going to see eye to eye on things. We've had two serious discussions toward the end of summer where the question is, 'Are we going to keep living together?' Both of us have really strong feelings about working things out and staying together. And both of us have major complaints

about the other person and how things have to change if we are going to be able to stay together.

"So it's a very complex picture right now, I think. It's hard as
hell for me to sort things out. My momentary . . . intuitive . . . emotional grasp of things tells me one thing . . . and other times I'm
thinking more logically . . . sometimes it's a mix. It's very hard.

"It's very hard. . . . The stress of my being sick and the potential of Jon's being sick, although he's not, is really *enormous*. And
not just in the enormity of the fact of it, but in that my being sick
and what that means for Jon having to be . . . you know, it can't be
50-50 in terms of who's making the effort, when one person can't
make so much of an effort. And that's unfair, but that's sort of the
rules of the game here."

The therapist then asked Jon to say why he was here, and he explained
how frustrated he was with their constant bickering and their seeming
inability to agree on anything at all.

THE FIRST ENACTMENT

The therapist asked the men to turn their chairs toward each other and
discuss the situation together. Watching the enactment, the therapist
and the team behind the mirror were immediately struck by the enormous contrast between the story of their early enchantment with each
other and the grim reality of daily life together now. Seth and Jon's bliss-
ful honeymoon phase was over. Where once the other's personality,
emotional style, and idiosyncratic behaviors were charming and appeal-
ing, they were now found to be irritating. The two partners seemed
locked in a struggle to change each other. But this couple was attempting to work out the details of a relationship precisely at a time when one
of them was also gravely ill. As John Rolland (1987) has described,
problems and symptoms of conflict often emerge when the course of
chronic illness intersects with the developmental needs of individuals,
couples, and families. With this couple, the developmental work of
accommodating to each other's needs while hanging onto one's individuality—a task all couples face in their early years together—was constrained by their mutual knowledge that one of them had full-blown
AIDS and might be dying. How could they make the necessary sacrifices

required in coming together as a couple when they knew fully well that one might soon die? They had barely worked out their routine for "normal times" when suddenly they were forced to contend with AIDS.

Rather than comment on their struggle to change each other and possibly begin an unbalancing maneuver, the therapist continued to join with the couple and collect more information. She learned that from day one they had had significant problems establishing a boundary around them as a couple. Both of their families continuously trespassed into their relationship. As Seth had recently become sicker with opportunistic infections, his mother had become more markedly intrusive. Jon's sister dropped by unannounced frequently and volunteered unsolicited advice to Jon on how to manage both Seth's illness and Seth's stoic personality. AIDS, in our experience, often exacerbates preexisting boundary issues for male couples as the extended family—often, only trying to be helpful—intrude (for good or ill) into the couple's business.

By the end of their first session, the couple had confided openly to the therapist about their issues and seemed fairly well joined with her. But, knowing they had expressed concerns about working with her, the supervisor encouraged the therapist to ask about their experience of her. The couple responded that they felt comfortable and wanted to continue with her. Taking a one-down position, the therapist suggested that, if they ever felt she was missing something about them as a gay couple, they should speak up and try to help her. They agreed. They asked the therapist whether she was in a relationship herself, and she answered candidly and simply that, in fact, she was taking some vacation soon to get married.[2]

MORE ENACTMENTS AND AN INITIAL UNBALANCING

At the next session the men came in fighting about Seth's mother, upset over her meddling in their relationship. She had visited that weekend from Philadelphia. Jon exclaimed angrily, "She just pushed me aside and took care of Seth herself!" Moreover, during the weekend Seth had

---

[2] When gay couples ask questions about the therapist's sexual orientation, we advocate answering honestly. The therapist can explore later what it means to the couple to be working with a therapist of the same or different sexual orientation, but the question itself deserves an immediate and truthful answer.

confided to his mother how much stress Jon was causing him. The finale to the mother's visit, as she was departing in a cab to catch her train back to Philadelphia, was pulling Jon aside and asking him to move out. She pleaded with Jon, "Just leave! Please leave! You are causing my son so much distress."

The therapist listened patiently and silently to their report of the weekend. Then she unbalanced the couple's customary dynamic by simply asking them, "Do you really need your families to give you so much advice on how to run your relationship? Or maybe your primary loyalty is, after all, to your families? Can you decide this issue here, right now? Who comes first for each of you?"

The men sat speechless and stunned. A successful unbalancing maneuver should, in fact, shake up the couple, disarming them in their tracks. With her intervention, the therapist seemed to be taking their relationship more seriously than they did. As the men sat in silence, the therapist asked them to talk together now about their competing loyalties to each other versus their families. After considerable dialogue, each concluded that his primary loyalty was to the other, but each admitted he had no idea about how to make sure his family understood this.

The therapist said she thought they needed a "bubble" around them to keep out the intruders. The couple grasped the "bubble" concept quickly and promised in the future not to involve family members in their issues as a couple. Knowing that promises weren't enough, the supervisor called in from behind the mirror and encouraged the therapist to create more intensity about this serious boundary issue.

The therapist said she herself was shocked that a parent would ask her son's partner to move out. Her use of self in this way invited the men to express their own feelings about having their couplehood disparaged by Seth's mother. Jon talked about how he had been hurt by Seth's mother's request that he should move out. As Jon became less angry and revealed his hurt, Seth took some responsibility for the incident by admitting that he had told her too much about their problems as a couple. The therapist urged Seth to make clear to his mother that Jon was his life partner and also his primary caretaker. Over the next month, Seth had several conversations with his mother, during which he apologized for involving her in their own problems and explained to her firmly that Jon was his partner and would not be leaving.

As the therapy progressed, the therapist honed in on the couple's communication problems. She staged many enactments, asking Seth and Jon to talk together about whatever issue had come up for them, keeping herself at a middle distance so she could observe their interactional pattern. It soon became clear to the treatment team behind the mirror that Seth and Jon were enacting a classic pursuer–distancer complementarity. As Jon would try to discuss an issue with Seth, Seth would sit in silence, appearing to reflect on the topic, and then deliver, like a well-constructed press release with reasoned logic, his views. He didn't seem to know how to engage in a give-and-take dialogue with Jon. Such reluctance on Seth's part to engage with him made Jon very impatient, so Jon frequently interrupted Seth's long-winded monologues, simply as a way to get Seth to connect with him, but a move that irritated Seth and pushed him further away. As he desperately tried to get Seth's attention, Jon would talk with his arms, amplifying his voice and facial expressions as he exaggerated his points for dramatic effect. Seth observed Jon's histrionics in stony silence, always staying composed but not knowing what to say or do next.

MORE UNBALANCING

The supervisor called the therapist to come talk with the team behind the mirror. After observing an enactment, it is critical to provide the couple with a frame—a mental image or a perspective—that captures what the therapist has seen. This aspect of learning structural family therapy can be further facilitated when the therapist has live supervision or is videotaping the sessions, because often it is difficult for the therapist to pull herself out of the content of what she is listening to and focus instead on nonverbal, interactional, and complementary dynamics. Such factors as these may be more easily perceived from behind the mirror or in watching the videotape after the session. As they gain greater experience, structural therapists learn to respond creatively to enactments more spontaneously in session.

After consulting with the team, the therapist returned to the consultation room and told the men that she and the team were in shock. "It's like both of you are from difficult cultures and speak different languages. It's absolutely amazing. What country is each of you from?" Each man then talked about where and how he had been raised. Seth described being influenced by a southern WASP ethic in which he had learned to be emotionally restrained and always logical. Emotional intensity frightened him. He believed instead in stoic self-reliance. He said he liked being with people but admitted that he needed lots of solitude. It was solitude that restored him. Always polite, he would go out of his way to please others, sometimes to his own detriment. The idea that two people might disagree and remain connected was alien to him, and he admitted he didn't know how to handle conflict. He said he simply froze when confronted with conflict.

Jon said growing up in a large Jewish family in the Bronx had taught him to speak up and "to take people on." He had learned to be feisty. He liked social interaction and welcomed emotional intensity. He didn't mind conflict. Seth's long silences and emotional withdrawal made Jon crazy with frustration. At home, Jon literally followed Seth from room to room to force some interaction. Seth would eventually retreat to the bedroom and shut the door, saying he needed his privacy and his rest.[3]

Introducing humor by tagging their complementary emotional styles as the WASP way and the Jewish way (since the men had put these stereotypical labels on themselves), the therapist began interrupting their fights, unbalancing the men by saying suddenly, "Oh, I see, Jon is trying to make Seth Jewish today! Would Seth's mother want him to convert?"

The therapist encouraged the men to educate each other about their respective cultures and emotional styles. She insisted each needed to translate his customs and his language, and, moreover, as a couple to begin to form their own blended culture in a new household. While the therapist acknowledged and accepted each man's native emotional style, she pushed the couple to accommodate each other's style.

"You live in one country now and must develop a common language," she told them. She prompted Seth to explain to Jon how to recognize the signs when a normally sedate, polite WASP was upset. She coached Jon at times to "stop being a Jewish mother" and give Seth more autonomy. The therapist's Jewish–WASP metaphor "grafted" onto

---

[3] In terms of attachment theory, we might say that Seth is more an "insecure/anxious" subtype who is accustomed to distancing in close relationships, whereas Jon is more an "insecure/ambivalent" subtype who needs greater closeness in relationships and becomes anxious when the partner appears too distant.

the couple, and they were soon able to catch themselves when they were trying to change the other to behave differently.

By the end of 4 months of treatment, the couple had been helped to dialogue more effectively with each other, to resolve several specific issues where they were in conflict, and to put a much firmer boundary around themselves as a couple. When one or the other, seeking an ally, would try to draw the therapist into their fights, she calmly demurred. Maintaining her middle distance, she would simply motion with her hands for the men to deal with each other directly. She continued to challenge each man on his step in the complementary dance they did together. At times, highlighting their enactments, she chided Jon that his incessant chatter left no airspace for Seth, and wondered aloud if Seth had stopped talking because Jon talked far more than he listened. At other times, she challenged Seth about the loneliness of the WASP way—and couldn't he find a way to make contact with Jon? Slowly, the couple's fighting decreased, talk of splitting up ended altogether, and the couple became much more satisfied with their relationship. Fortunately, for much of this time, Seth's health was stable.

Then, in late December, Seth again began having serious medical problems. He was diagnosed with Kaposi's sarcoma. The couple came in fighting over how to manage Seth's declining energy level. The following verbatim transcript illustrates how well the men had learned "to stay in the room" when in conflict with each other. This particular exchange is also interesting for its content, as it describes fundamental differences in how people cope with debilitating illness. For Seth and Jon, the ways they coped with illness reflected their own individual emotional styles.

JON: The only problem I have with our relationship now is that he's sick. There is no other problem. I mean . . . we're actually doing pretty well, considering all of what's going on. We're rather happy with each other.

SETH: Yeah, but it's the other issues that are attendant to my being sick that we've got on the table right now, isn't it?

THERAPIST: What are you thinking about?

SETH: Where the discussion was before we came in here today . . .

JON: It's in my head right now that discussion. And I'm thinking that at this second . . .

THERAPIST: What discussion?

JON: That I push him out . . . I had done that in the past . . .

THERAPIST: That you push him out? Oh, you push him *to go out.*

JON: That had been true in the past. . . . That's absolutely true. But that has not been true this week. He's been sick for so long that . . . you know, it's like . . . I get it now.

SETH: I think I may have misread the signals from Jon. When he said, you know, try to get up . . . look, you're feeling well, let's try to enjoy this time, this is the good time again.

JON: That's exactly what I said, but that didn't mean going out!

SETH: I know, honey, but I'm not a totally logical person. Because of history and because of my need to not have you upset and panicked about me, I've been really trying to be . . . more up and more vigorous about doing things.

And I wasn't saying, Jon pushed me. I was saying I pushed myself in response to what I thought was happening. Now, I am not holding you responsible, but I'm holding us . . . as the patterns that we've set up, as least as responsible as I am holding me personally. Now I'm 40 years old. . . . This is one of the things I'm not so good

Seth has begun to think like a systems therapist! His comments reflect his growing insight that their problems as a

at in my life, not overvaluing other people's needs as they express themselves to me and putting it into my planning. I have always done that . . . like, knocked myself out to get something done for somebody and it turns out it wasn't really important for them.

THERAPIST: I think you both do that, don't you?

SETH: I've really wanted to do everything I can for you. . . . This has been an incredibly stressful time. I knew it was stressful with my mother coming. And the kids had been maniacs at school. So I was really trying, and . . .

JON: He wrapped 28 presents [for the school kids]!!!!

    Seth, you are always trying; you're a wonderful spouse and companion. I never say you're not.

SETH: No, but bad things sometimes happen out of good intentions. That's all I'm saying, I'm not trying to make you feel bad because I got pushed. . . . I'm trying to make sure that we outline the issue enough so that sometime when I'm not doing so well and really am trying, that we've covered this.

JON: We've been over this 100 times. This is a . . .

SETH: No! Last week was the first time we ever . . .

JON: This is a fundamental difference in perspective. It's not I don't get the outline. I'm not a moron! It is a fundamental difference in perspective. I honestly feel that

couple are not because of just one of them, but that they are caught up in interactional patterns. The therapist has succeeded in expanding the couple's thinking.

life is about . . . doing things!! Interfacing with people, saying hello to people, chatting people up, going to the dry cleaners, this is the stuff of life!

(Phone rings with input from the supervisor.)

THERAPIST: Seth, it's a really important question how Jon is going to handle it when you get sick and have to go to the hospital . . . and when you're not so active. I think it does deserve an answer.

Jon, can you talk to Seth about how you are going to be?

JON: I feel I just answered that question.

THERAPIST: *(to Seth)* Did you feel Jon answered it? . . . Do you know how he's going to be?

SETH: He said, essentially, he'll cope with it when he has to. That's what I heard.

THERAPIST: Let's talk about the details now. Because not talking about it doesn't keep it from happening. It's going to happen, and planning for it will make it less stressful and less "crisisy" when it does, and it will relieve the pressure that you both feel now. So . . . Talk about the details of what it's going to be like.

JON: You mean, when he goes to the hospital? . . . I don't know how to answer this question! I mean, what will happen? I'll go everyday! . . . I'll sit there. I'll try to do what I can do to make his life easier in the hospital.

THERAPIST: *(to Seth)* Is the question "How is Jon going to be emotionally?" What part do you want answered the most?

A spontaneous enactment is beginning here, reflecting again the dynamics of the couple. But the dialogue is beginning to lose focus, so the supervisor asks the therapist to help the couple focus on the one issue that seems so difficult to confront.

The tendency to avoid talking about the worst-case scenario in end-of-life issues only raises anxiety for the family. With gentle encouragement, the therapist sets up an enactment that encourages the men to talk about this difficult issue more directly.

The therapist creates intensity by helping the couple nail down the issue even more sharply.

SETH: Well, the origin of the question was really about . . . like I have only a certain
amount of being able to rise above things.
And I've always had a lot of it. But I'm
not having that much flexibility in my
physical response now. . . . I'm just concerned about the pattern between us
when Jon sees me resting. I thought, in a
way, the question is getting at a "If you lie
down, you're dead" philosophy. (*to Jon*)
When I lie down, somehow in your mind
I'm dead.

(*Silence*)

JON: I feel you need to get out!! You need to
have a life!! You need to be a part of the
world of the living. When you're in the
hospital, you can't participate in that way,
but I'll figure out other ways for you to
participate. But you are not in the hospital
now. Now!

This is my way. He likes his mother's
way. (*Speaking to the team behind the one-
way mirror*) Sorry, I know I'm not supposed to . . . This is the truth of it: His
mother's way is: He says, "I want to lay
here," and she says, "OK, let me sit and
hold your hand." That's OK, she's his
mother. That's not my way, that's not what
I want to give him. Not now. He's not sick
enough for that, and I won't give him
that.

(*Now really worked up, Jon pauses to
catch his breath.*) If he doesn't feel up to
it, he should be able to say, "I don't feel
up to it." And like not judge me for
thinking . . . I know he's not really up to
it. But I want to give him the offer any-
way. It's like . . .

THERAPIST: You want to be helpful.

JON: Because I want him to feel like . . .

SETH: I'm alive.

And the scary part is that it's probably a middle path. It's good for me to get up and out, and it's also good for me not to. And I hate to feel I'm always the one who's deciding not to do things . . .

JON: Honey, it's your health. You have to make the decision. I can't.

SETH: I know. I'm not talking about rational. I'm saying I hate to feel . . .

THERAPIST: Aside from that, and because I know you will work that out and I'll help you with that, but I am wondering (*to Jon*) about your feelings, too, and whether Seth can help with your feelings, hold you and comfort you . . .

JON: I can't even think about that . . . I have waited my whole life for this. I can't . . . I can't . . .

This is the first time I feel like I'm a part of something. My mother died when I was 8 years old, this is my first real family. My own family. My own home. My own life. I can't imagine a life without Seth. I've waited so long for him, and . . . I'm so sad that my love can't make him. . . . (*crying*) But my sister keeps telling me to get him out of the house. I think she's right.

THERAPIST: Your sister??

SETH: I didn't know that.

THERAPIST: Can we leave your sister also out? (*to Seth*) How do you help Jon with what he's feeling, he's saying that it's such

When a couple is fighting over a specific issue, it is tempting for the therapist to take sides or to help them find a compromise. Here the therapist stays out of the issue altogether and instead asks each man to help the other.

The therapist helps the men maintain boundaries and avoid

a gift to have you? It's hard for him to lose you.

SETH: It seems to me that . . . many times Jon's responses are relatively influenced not by the brain but by the heart. And the panic that comes up or the sense of urgency about things. Sometimes it's good to be pushed, and sometimes it's good not to be pushed. The middle path . . . sometimes it's good to really luxuriate in not pushing at all, and just lie around.

JON: Let me be clear: I don't want you to die and me to feel that my pushing killed you. I'll kill myself. I really want to be clear about this. It's very important. And I also feel you need to get out!! You need to get out; I feel you can't sit around all the time. You can't atrophy, you need to get out!

You have to be with people. That's why I'm always making dinner, why I'm inviting people . . . why do you think I'm always inviting people over? So that you have people over, so that I have people over, so that we interface with other people, we're still interesting! Let's . . . you know!!

So you can say "I can't do it, maybe tomorrow," and not judge like I don't know where you're coming from. Believe me, I know what's going on for you. It's not that I don't know. It's that I think maybe you'll feel better if you do something, you'll feel more aliveness if you do something. If you don't want to do it, I don't want you to do it.

I always want to offer you aliveness rather than sickness.

triangulating Jon's sister. The therapist keeps them on track to deal with what is happening to them emotionally as a couple, specifically, Jon's fear of losing Seth.

SETH: This is where what you're intending and what I'm feeling is so different. To me, spending two days in bed means that I may have five good days after it. If I can recharge my batteries enough when I feel like lying down, I can get up from it refreshed . . . which is how it worked the last time I was sick, so sick I just had to stay in bed for days. Well, I got better!

I didn't get better by having so many people come over and talk to me; I got better by resting! This is a foreign concept to you.

You don't see that as progress, whereas I see that if I rest up when my vaguest inclination is to rest, then I am putting money in the bank.

The men themselves have taken up the therapist's metaphor that they are from different cultures and speak different languages. Thus, the therapist's frame has now grafted. The couple is at the cusp of discovering the third language of "we" that bridges the two cultures.

JON: Well, my mother died with a needle and thread in her hand, sewing a Hanukkah menorah thing for me. I feel people keep working . . . you keep doing things!

SETH: This is where we are speaking different languages.

THERAPIST: Is it OK if you have different ideas of how to live? Is that all right?

JON: It's OK, but I have to do what I have to do to keep him well. It's so confusing to me, it's like . . . what if he's wrong and I'm right?

FINAL SESSION OF COUPLE TREATMENT

For the next 6 weeks, the couple was unable to come for their regular sessions. Seth became seriously ill and was hospitalized for 3 weeks. The therapist stayed in phone contact with the couple. In late January Seth was discharged, but he was too weak to come to the clinic for a couple session. The couple called to ask the therapist to make a home visit to their apartment, which she did. Here is an example of how the boundaries of traditional therapy can become more flexible when working with the terminally ill.

In late February the couple called the therapist with some urgency to request a session with the team behind the mirror. Jon would arrange for Seth to be brought to the clinic by ambulette. Jon explained that the doctors didn't expect Seth to regain his health and that Seth had decided he wanted to die at home. They were having a difficult time making arrangements and managing their anxiety.

Seth arrived at the clinic in a wheelchair and was connected to a morphine drip. Because Seth had held in his arms his previous lover as he died, had found that experience very fulfilling, and thought it had also been consoling to his dying lover, it was now his desire to die the same way. As the session began, around 4 o'clock, the couple was discussing Jon's anxiety about Seth's plan for Jon to hold him in his arms as he was dying.

Unbeknownst, of course, to the therapist and the team, Seth would die at 8 o'clock that evening.

SETH: I'm right here, I have a big morphine patch on my shoulder, and my eyelids are going to droop. But I'm right here.

JON: (*crying, talking to therapist*) I can't imagine what my life is going to be like when he's gone. I try to make a picture with my head; I can't make a picture . . . I can't see it. And I keep thinking there's going to come the time that he's not going to be there, that he's going to be gone, and I'm probably going to be by myself.

This is really scary for me. And I want to do it [to have Seth die at home in his arms], but I don't want to do it by myself, I think. Maybe someone should be around. Kathy said she could be around, all I have to do is call her. She's a nurse.

THERAPIST: Well, can you talk to Seth about how he can help you?

At this point, it's not clear to anyone the extent to which Seth can participate in the session. But the therapist decides to ask Jon to engage Seth in the discussion.

JON: This is my question . . . I don't know
exactly. That's why I got so upset when he
was nodding out, maybe he can't help me.
Maybe it's too late.

THERAPIST: Well, why don't you ask? Seth
says he's been through this. Maybe he has
some ideas.

JON: Seth, do you have ways to help me with
this?

SETH: Well . . . there are a couple of things
going on. One is the question of your being afraid to be with my remains after I've
gone, and that's separate from being afraid
to be with me during the process of dying. I'm not sure I can help you with the
remains part . . . because it's not me anymore, and I'm not going to be there to
help you with it. Yet, it's still me.

    And I know the impulse to reach
down to hold a hand, to kiss the lips
the last time. But you know we are
two doors from Carpenter's [a funeral
home]. It's not going to be 1½ hours,
like it was for me; it's going to be 15
minutes.

    And it's going to be . . . agony, and
then you'll wish you had more. You
know? These are my thoughts on that
part of it.

JON: So . . . when you're dying and not able
to talk to me, what are the things you'd
want to say, maybe you can say them now.

SETH: I think you know them all, you know
them all by heart, honey. It's all about
how much I love you. And how grateful I
am for your love, your willingness to go
through the deepest nightmares of your
life to see me through . . . this process. It's

*Discipline for the
therapist is required
when the family is
working well. For the
next few minutes,
both therapist and
supervisor are entirely
quiet as they observe
the couple deeply
engage each other in
dialogue.*

all of that stuff, and . . . I say it to you
now and I'll say it to you again and again,
and you're going to hear me saying it to
you even if I'm not saying anything, that's
what you'll hear echoing.

JON: This is really exactly what I'm talking
about. I have no question that you love
me. Huh! This is not, you know, like
something I question or I doubt or I fear.
I'm crystal clear about that, but . . .

SETH: What are you asking me?

JON: I'm not asking you to tell me you love
me. I know you love me. I'm asking you
to tell me . . .

SETH: You're asking me what will I say to
you that I won't be able to say, and I'm
telling you.

JON: That you love me.

SETH: That's not all I said, but yes. Don't reduce it all like that, honey.

JON: See, I really know that, if you could . . .
that . . . you would stay. But I also know
that you can't really stay, but . . . I really
do believe that if you could, you would.
That's how much you love me.

SETH: Is that what you want to hear me say?

JON: I want you to hear you say that. I want
to feel that you're going because you have
no other choice . . .

SETH: OH! Hmmmm . . .

JON: . . . not because I've done something
wrong, or I didn't take good enough care
of you, or maybe I pushed you too much.

SETH: Now I'm hearing it. I'm hearing it.
Don't be scared of that. Honey, we're be-

yond that. You're beyond that. I'm beyond that. This is . . .

This is about inevitability.

This is about . . . my worn-out body and the balance that I find between comfort and the time I can spend with you.

JON: Seth, just tell me, please, just tell me that you wouldn't leave if you didn't have to, please . . .

SETH: Of course I wouldn't leave if I didn't have to leave! Do you think . . . what do you think? It's so . . .

THERAPIST: Say it a couple more times. Seth, say it a couple more times, so Jon can hear you.

The therapist's goal here was to intensify Seth's statement so that Jon could "take it in."

SETH: I'm not leaving because of anything you've done. All right? There is nothing you have done or left undone that is making me leave. There is nothing that you have done that is making me want to leave. There is nothing you have done that is making me leave.

(*Pause*)

You know . . . you're not 8 years old, you're a grown-up. You can get it from me: I'm telling you the God's honest truth: I'm not leaving because I want to; I'm leaving because it's inevitable, and . . . and the inevitability of it is postponed by how much I love you and how much (*coughing*) you do for me.

It's not anything that you've done that makes me want to leave; it's what you've done that makes me want to stay!!

JON: I love you so much. (*sobbing*) I just can't believe how . . . much I love you.

In a remarkable moment of deep empathy, Seth senses that Jon's reaction to Seth's death is related to what happened with his mother when he was 8. How powerful it is when this kind of insight and empathic understanding can come from one's partner. In this way, couple therapy can be

SETH: Do you really hear me?

JON: I really hear you.

SETH: OK.

transformational for one or both individuals.

(*A minute or two of silence*)

I feel that I want to tell that 8-year-old boy that it was exactly the same with your mother. She wanted to stay with you so badly, and she couldn't.

And it was nothing you did. You were a good little boy. And you've been a good partner and lover and . . . you've done everything you can for me, and I'd want to stay with you forever but I can't . . . I just can't. It's not because of anything you've done. It's because of . . . the facts . . . OK?

Seth begins to provide Jon with a healing conversation he wasn't able to have with his own mother.

(*Silence for a few moments*)

JON: You'll see my mother . . . (*crying*) and she'll see you.

SETH: And she'll say, thank you for telling him I didn't want to leave him . . .

And you know, she had a lot of people she was leaving, her husband, three daughters, you, her sisters, her mother.

I've got you that I'm leaving, honey. You . . . you're my focus.

Jon takes in what Seth has said and expands it.

JON: And your mother . . .

SETH: My mother hates the fact that I'm dying, but it's not about my leaving her in her mind the way it is with you.

JON: If I could explain it to you . . . This is how much I love you . . . that when I met you, I knew that this would be the end . . . of our relationship. And I loved you so much that I was willing to face this, and now I'm so scared. But that's how much I loved you.

I never thought I could feel this much about anyone . . . except . . . well, maybe, my dog . . . but . . . it's like . . . it's like I want to make sure that when the time comes I will do it right, and I'm clear, that my shit's not in the way, and that I don't call someone to come because I'm nervous. . . . It's like I'd rather do it myself.

SETH: You know what? I . . . I . . . I . . . I honestly believe that it's not going to be . . . I don't have a strong feeling that you need to tough it out . . . to be there by yourself. You know, . . . if it helps you . . . if I'm on a morphine drip and on my way out, have Patricia [Jon's friend] there, have your sister there. It's really OK.

I'm going to be on the way out, and . . . there's nothing more that I will be able to do for you, and I'd be so grateful if there's someone who can do something for you.

(Phone rings from the supervisor.)

THERAPIST: Hmmm . . . you know . . . we want to say thank you, because the team is really very moved . . . about what you've been able to talk about today.

I mean . . . I just feel extraordinarily grateful to be able to see so much love. I don't know if I've ever felt my heart so full, to see how the two of you care for each other in the way that you do, and you saying what you said to Jon about wanting to stay . . . it's just . . .

SETH: I just wasn't getting what you were asking of me. I'm sorry I was being dense.

JON: You caught on awfully fast.

When the therapist witnesses such an authentic exchange between a couple, it is important to reflect back what she has seen, to reveal how moved she was by it, and to highlight how different it was from the couple's past conversations. In addition, the therapist can acknowledge that the couple's profound connection to each other

THERAPIST: It just says how much you've grown as a couple, how quickly you do catch on.

   Why don't we end it there? I, and the team, will be thinking of you. Will we see you next week?

(*The supervisor enters the consultation room.*)

SUPERVISOR: (*to Seth*) We couldn't believe you were nodding out at all. It sounds like you've got all the burners going today.

SETH: Thank you.

SUPERVISOR: I don't know whether I've ever witnessed like this.

   (*to Seth*) And I think you are taking care of him right up until the last minute.

JON: I think so too.

SUPERVISOR: Everything you were saying . . . you were saying everything this man needed to hear, and I hope you heard it, especially the part about being 8. I hope you heard it.

JON: I did.

SETH: I know this 8-year-old. I married him.

SUPERVISOR: If you two can't make it next week . . . I don't want you to feel obligated. It took an enormous effort for you to get here today.

SETH: It was well worth it.

JON: We really like to do it.

SUPERVISOR: I know, but (*to Jon*) you have a lot of guilt . . . about a lot of things . . . and I don't want this to become one of those things. That if you say you're coming in and then you can't come, I don't

has also made her feel more connected to them as a couple.

The therapist gives the couple credit and reinforces how they have changed.

The supervisor decided to enter the room from behind the mirror to emphasize again what he and the treatment team had witnessed.

In retrospect, the supervisor must have sensed that afternoon that it was probably the last time he would see Seth and Jon as a couple, and it was important to make personal contact one last time.

want you to feel that you are letting us down. Are we clear about that?

JON: Yes, but I want you to be clear. This hour is one of the most important hours of our lives. So, we really want to be here.

SUPERVISOR: So the hour is yours if you can come.

Weeks later, Jon told the therapist that working with her and the team had made them feel for the first time in their lives "validated" as a couple.

The next morning the therapist received a call from Jon that Seth had died that night, 3 hours after the session. He had died at home in Jon's arms.

The therapist offered Jon an individual session the next day, but he was busy making funeral arrangements. In a few days he called to invite the therapist and the treatment team, whom he had never met, to attend Jon's memorial service, which they did. The therapist saw Jon for several individual sessions to talk about the details of Seth's death and his own grief. In one session, she asked Jon if he'd like a copy of the video-tape of their last couple's session together. Jon asked his rabbi to watch it with him, an experience that seemed to legitimize further their couplehood.

In his final meeting alone with the therapist, Jon told her that just that morning when he was putting away dinner plates, he had found a handwritten note from Seth under the ninth plate. The note read, "Well, if you are down to using this many dinner plates, it means you are back to entertaining and living again. I'm glad."

DISCUSSION

Before the final session, this couple's therapy would have been regarded as successful by most family therapists. Jon and Seth had been helped to place a firmer boundary around their relationship, they had learned to manage conflict, they had become more tolerant of each other's emotional style, they had learned to accommodate each other's needs, and they had become more content with their relationship. But it was the final session that transformed them and started us thinking, some 10 years ago, about what is sometimes missing in work with male couples.

In their last meeting with their therapist, Seth and Jon became a couple authentically engaged with each other. Their dialogue, on the precipice of a partner's death, is very poignant. Over the years it has become especially meaningful to us that *this dialogue took place between two men*. We think that is all too rare. What were the conditions that made it happen? Was it possible only because one of the partners was dying? We don't think that's the primary reason they spoke so directly to each other.

For one thing, not all couples, straight or gay, become closer emotionally on the cusp of serious illness and dying. Wide variability exists in how families cope with illness and death (Rolland, 1994), and life-threatening illness is a time when family members often become more estranged and distant rather than closer. Couples who already have good connectedness often become even closer during times of stress. Couples who are more disconnected in normal times become even more so during stressful times. Although Seth and Jon bickered a lot, they were nonetheless strongly attached to each other prior to Seth's becoming so ill. Their mutual caring for each other never wavered—even when they fought bitterly.

Instead of disconnecting as death closed in on them, as a result of their therapy Seth and Jon became even more connected to each other, stopped their bickering, dropped their defensive armor, and were able to be astonishingly present for each other. Their final dialogue in couple treatment was a tough one to have, yet they persevered in having it. We think the primary reason they were able to have it was that the 7 months of therapy had created a greater sense of "we-ness." They had learned that they could count on each other to be responsive to their needs. It also seemed important that the team behind the mirror was somehow serving as a community that gave validity to the gay couple's relationship, providing the one safe place that accepted them fully as a couple.

During their last meeting the couple indelibly imprinted upon us the healing potential of an emotionally connecting experience for gay men, who generally learn during their early years how to face life alone. Seth and Jon demonstrated how males—despite their façade of separateness and stoic independence—are not emotionally vacant, but under the right conditions can forge incredibly strong emotional connections. Seth and Jon taught us about empathic attunement between men, and how a connecting experience with another man can be psychologically healing. Seth, through his profound empathy for Jon, just hours before his own death helped Jon to heal a deep-rooted sense of abandonment, a wound that had festered since childhood. Jon never had a chance to tell his mother good-bye, and his mother never was able to tell him that he had been a good son and was in no way responsible for her death. The loss of his primary attachment figure when he was 8 had made him particularly vulnerable to separation and loss, and impacted on his initial emotional reaction to Seth's impending death: he had wanted Seth to keep going, to stay active and socially involved, not to give in to illness and death by prematurely retiring from life, which his "lying down" had come to symbolize for Jon. In the December session Jon was not ready to give Seth up.

By the final session in February Jon understood what they were facing. Seth was indeed dying. All of Jon's old issues of abandonment emerged full force. Seth knew what those issues were, and he, in an incredible expression of compassion and empathy, connected the dots for Jon. He understood that Jon's reaction to his dying—that Jon was somehow to blame—was related to his having lost his mother when he was only 8. Seth gave Jon a precious gift, namely, that his partner could understand him emotionally to the core. The dialogue with Seth became a corrective emotional experience for Jon.

It is noteworthy that in the last session, when Seth is dying, that he does not discuss his own feelings about dying. In his characteristic way he is looking out for someone else and putting the other's needs over his own. He remained emotionally self-reliant and fairly stoic in terms of his own personal needs. Perhaps helping his partner confront and master his old demons gave Seth an inner peace just before dying, that his work was now indeed done. Although Seth never asks Jon for help in talking about his impending death, he does make a very special request of his partner. He does not want to die alone; he wants Jon to hold him in his arms. Could Seth really be a stoic distancer if he can make such a

request?! This is a dramatic example of a structural family therapy axiom that connectedness isn't just verbal. That is, individuals may or may
not have adequate vocabulary to verbalize their emotional connectivity,
but they can find other ways to communicate it.

Rarely have we seen men in therapy so emotionally attuned to each
other in the way Seth and Jon were. During the years since their treatment we have sought to understand how they were able to do this in
that last session, that is, to stay close together, to remain in the moment
where they were about to lose each other and yet feel so connected to
each other. Impending death may have had something to do with it,
but, as we have noted, many couples avoid emotional connection at a
time of imminent loss. We think, in retrospect, the couple's empathic
attunement in their last session can be attributed to the therapist's interventions in that final session. She evidenced an ability to stay with the
couple's intense affect, not to flinch from it but to bear it along with
them. Her facilitating style in that particular session—her trust that, if
she stayed at the periphery, the two men would find the resources to
lovingly help each other—allowed them to have a profound conversation that led to a strong empathic connection. For us, the pivotal moment in the session came when Seth, struggling to understand what it
was that Jon needed him to say, "gets it." It is a moment of real empathy
of "we-ness" as a couple: Seth steps out of himself, puts himself in Jon's
shoes, and has an emotional understanding of his partner.

Did the therapist's being female somehow help these two men
make connection? The thought has crossed our mind, given that it is a
cultural belief that women are better able to create and maintain connectedness. The supervisor has from time to time felt that if he, a southern-
raised male with a WASP background, had been the therapist in that
final session, he might have done something to have cut off the intense
affect—not because the men were having a hard time with it, but because *he* was! Fortunately, he didn't call in from behind the one-way
mirror and suggest WASPish emotional restraint. Instead, from behind
the one-way mirror on February 23, 1993, he with the four other psychology interns watched a therapist holding these men's feelings, sitting
with her own while crying at times along with the men, managing her
own ambiguity about what was transpiring and instead following the
couple's lead, and not being afraid of the intensely sad affect in the
room. The therapist's interventions were minimal but profound. Through-

out the final session, she continuously asks each man to help the other emotionally. What a revolutionary idea: helping two men take care of each other emotionally!

Since this case, we more routinely push male couples to make emotional contact. The case began a fundamental change in the goal in treating male couples—emphasizing emotional connective work between the men, helping them develop, maintain, and honor their attachment to each other. Within our overall structural family model, we push gay men to become more affectively attuned to each other. Many of the unbalancing interventions discussed in this volume have had this as their goal: for men to lay down their guns and begin to experiment with expressing loving, tender, and vulnerable feelings in the presence of another man, and for the other to respond supportively.

CHAPTER EIGHT

Toward the Future

As we were completing this chapter, one of us was consulting from behind a one-way mirror, observing an initial therapy session in which a family was reacting to the news that an older child, 27, was gay. The family had come for therapy because the preadolescent daughter was persistently vomiting every morning to avoid going to school. As it turned out, her 27-year-old brother, Greg, who still lived at home with the family and was especially close to his sister, had told her several weeks before that he was gay and had a boyfriend. Greg also had asked his sister not to reveal the secret to their parents. The girl had been put in an awful bind, wanting to honor her brother's request yet unable to manage the brother's revelation on her own. Greg's news had upset her personally, plus she feared her parents' reactions once they found out. The girl was literally throwing up because she couldn't contain information that was difficult, even toxic, to her. Based on what she had heard at church about homosexuality and knowing her parents were deeply religious, she feared specifically that the parents would throw her brother out of the house. Although she was angry with Greg, she didn't want to lose him.

As the family talked, it turned out that the parents, while initially shocked and disappointed by the news that their son was gay, were also tolerant and were prepared to accept the son's homosexuality. Unbeknownst to the younger child until the family session, the father's daughter from a previous marriage, Janet, now 34, and someone whom the younger child was close to, was also homosexual. The father had maintained a very strong, loving relationship with Janet and announced during the session that he planned to do the same with Greg. The mother had known all along of her stepdaughter's homosexuality and had not been especially bothered by it. But now she was struggling with accepting her own son's gayness, an experience that seemed quite different to her. She worried aloud in the session whether she, having a son who had "turned" gay, could ever return to her church. The mother's embarrassment and shame was palpable.

The entire family is now in the process of slowly working through their acceptance of the son's homosexuality. The odds are strong that the father won't disown him, the mother will return to her church, and the younger daughter's love for her big brother will return. But, we ask, is this scenario as good as it gets for gay people?

This family is loving and supportive. Yet, listening to the parents and the younger child speak about homosexuality in the session reminded us just how homophobic the culture remains. Their words stung. The father spoke of his guilt in having *two* gay children. He was convinced he must have done something wrong. He said, "You know, some children turn out to be drug dealers and prostitutes. Despite my children's lifestyles, I still love them." The mother said, "I am so ashamed. My son's behavior is a sin and goes against God." The younger child spoke of her anger at her brother for "choosing" such a "disgusting" lifestyle. She asked, "What if my friends ever find out?"

Now that Greg's secret is out, the family needs time to digest the new information and vent their feelings. And, as we have said, in all likelihood they will end up accepting Greg back into the fold, just as they previously had accepted Janet. However, it is sad to us that this sort of begrudging acceptance is often considered a good outcome by gay people and by many therapists. The family's acceptance is beyond tolerance, but it seems qualified at best, most likely leaving their gay children feeling marginalized or "less than." We can only imagine what Greg and Janet, who weren't present at the initial family session, have experienced in hiding their secrets and in what remarks they heard while coming out to the family. We wonder when the day will come where the news that a family member is gay is not immediately met with revulsion, shock, anger, shame, and guilt. Will the day ever come when being gay is accepted just as easily as being left-handed? Probably not, at least not in our lifetime.

On the other hand, attitude change on a societal level can happen, though it is a tediously slow process. It usually always starts with one

person, one couple, one family. We think our model is a good beginning. Our model respects and honors the male couple's relationship. In
valuing it, we convey to the couple that it is worth preserving and is
worth working on. Moreover, we challenge the men to make it better, to
forge stronger emotional bonds to each other, and to reduce their "relational ambiguity" (Green & Mitchell, 2002). As the men begin to
change their views toward themselves in our consulting rooms, they return to the real world often radiating a new respect for their relationship. Their family and community can see that and perhaps begin to
question their own negative attitudes and beliefs toward gay men and
their relationships. But such societal change must start with the couple
itself.

In several of the case studies presented in this volume, at times we
found ourselves taking the couple's relationship more seriously than the
couple did. Their lack of respect toward their own relationship mirrors
the culture's views toward same-sex relationships. When a therapist
takes a male couple seriously by validating their relationship, the couple is started down a path toward having a corrective experience in how
they feel about themselves. By our actively respecting their relationship
in the earliest stages of treatment, we help them experience their relationship as legitimate and valuable.

Our therapy isn't just about supporting or protecting the couple
from the homophobia of the culture. Our therapy, like the structural
family therapy model on which it is based, is distinctive from other
models of therapy in that it is based on challenge. We say implicitly to
the couple, "You can do better." The challenge begins in the very first
session. A couple almost always casts its problems in individual terms.
Individuals may point their fingers at each other in blame, or one may
cite a unique history in defense of himself that communicates that he
really can't be any different. We don't readily accept individual-based
psychopathology. As systemic family therapists, we believe individual
problems are *interpersonal* in origin.

Following that belief, we focus on the couple's immediate interpersonal context. It is in the here-and-now interactional context, occurring
in front of the therapist, that their problems will be acted out. And it is
in this same immediate context where the therapeutic action concen-
trates. Thus, usually in the first session, our model begins expanding
the problem from a focus on the individual to a focus on the couple. As
the couple first speak about their problems, either insinuating or force-

fully charging that the other partner is at fault, we listen with a third ear and watch with our eyes for something else more important, namely, how has the couple structured itself? We put the couple's interactional context under a magnifying glass. If we look carefully, their relational structure will reveal itself in their moment-to-moment interaction with each other. The question at this stage of therapy is always the same: what is each individual doing to the other, in a repetitive, complementary fashion, that maintains their problems? The answer to this question becomes the map for the treatment.

This shift in focus from individual to system may expand a family's understanding of their problem. They may begin to have an intellectual appreciation of their respective roles in sustaining the problem, although many families fight back as we try to make that shift. Even if they "get it"—that is, understand how each is contributing to the problem in a pattern of complementarity—their insight is never sufficient for lasting change to occur. Insight may be interesting, but by itself it is not sufficient to create change. *The couple must be made to feel uncomfortable about what they are doing as they do it.* The couple must have an emotional experience that makes their current behavior feel dissonant.

Raising the level of emotional intensity for family members is a hallmark of the structural model. Unbalancing techniques are used to disrupt rigid, habitual patterns. A disruption must occur in a family's old, familiar grooves before the family can discover new resources and start to cut new grooves. Stated another way, if the main highway is blocked—once drivers get over their initial anxiety and anger—they almost always become more creative. They start discovering new routes. The structural model holds that all drivers are creative, and blocking old routes is one way to help them become more spontaneous and flexible.

Helping couples find new pathways produces anxiety in couples (and in family therapists). But without that anxiety, nothing much changes. We are asking clients to change highways, to leave the old paths they have become so familiar with, even when the paths are painful, difficult, or merely boring. Moreover, we don't find or impose the new routes on them! That creates even more tension. Although we may point them in the right direction, the couple really is in the driver's seat. As they begin exploring new paths, the therapist becomes a passenger in the car, enjoying the ride and continuing to do a little backseat driving from time to time.

Unbalancing in the structural model has the connotation of confrontation and direct challenge. However, unbalancing, as we have demonstrated, can consist of "soft" challenges as well as "hard" ones. The therapist in Chapter 7 is challenging, but her challenges are soft. She encourages the men to be more gentle with each other as they discuss their differences. Repeatedly in the final session, she asks one man to help the other manage what he is feeling. "Can you help him?" she repeatedly asks. For gay men, who are often shamed for being "soft," insisting that they be tender with their partner pushes them into a zone of discomfort.

What also makes our model distinctive and enriching for gay clients and therapists is a further expansion of the problem from the couple's system to the larger cultural contexts in which we all operate. Just as the presenting problem does not occur in one individual, the male couple does not exist isolated from its cultures, the mainstream culture into which each individual was born and the gay culture to which he has often developed some allegiance.

While our model never loses sight of the immediate interpersonal context surrounding the presenting problem, neither does it underestimate the potency of the mainstream culture in affecting how gay males develop as individuals and how they form and sustain long-term permanent partnerships. Male couples are affected enormously by mainstream culture in ways that impact on their own interpersonal dynamics. Despite the growing visibility of same-sex relationships, we remain by and large a homophobic society and a rather tightly gendered one. Individuals internalize the culture's attitudes about both homosexuality and gender, attitudes that on balance undermine long-term gay relationships.

During the late stages of treatment, the therapist often works with the couple to experience how cultural systems have constructed them and how they, wittingly or unwittingly, have played along. Because gay men get so little social support for their relationship and may settle for what little they get, they may inadvertently acquiesce in keeping their relationship invisible or marginal. They begin to experience how their culture—homophobic and rigidly gendered—has exacted its toll on their relationship, putting them in mental strait jackets (Green et al., 1996) in terms of what behaviors are considered possible. We help them examine the strait jackets and experiment with loosening or even removing them.

There is no question that tolerance by the mainstream culture of gay men and male couples has grown significantly during the past quarter-century. Some of these gains have been tangible. Large corporations now offer domestic partner benefits; some states make it easier for gay men and lesbians to adopt children; many states have legislation that includes sexual orientation in hate crimes; progressive schools teach an appreciation of nonstraight sexual orientation. In many ways gay people in the United States have never enjoyed a better time to be gay.

Despite such gains, discrimination against gay couples continues to be legal. Same-sex couples are not allowed to marry, and thus cannot take advantage of legal, economic, and social benefits that heterosexually married couples routinely enjoy. Gay couples attempting to build lifelong partnerships must go through elaborate financial planning processes that heterosexual couples do not have to face. Laws that discriminate in this way contribute to the instability of long-term gay relationships. The message from mainstream culture remains quite clear: not only are same-sex relationships different, they are most certainly "less than."

Finally, the other culture that impinges on the lives of male couples is the gay subculture. Because the mainstream culture makes gay men feel marginalized, the gay community has developed a certain culture of its own to combat the marginalization and to help gay men feel more bonded with one another. Although it doesn't have the rituals, customs, and values uniquely associated with a particular country or ethnic group, the gay subculture has nonetheless developed over the years certain traditions, tribal rites, and behaviors it considers normative, many of which attempt to create a sense of belonging. Gay bars and bathhouses developed, particularly after 1969, for men to meet, congregate, and feel connected to one another. In the last decade, circuit dance parties, Internet chat, and heavy use of recreational drugs (which create an artificial connectedness) have emerged to serve the same need: to help gay men feel less isolated. Fundamentally, the underlying need to belong and to connect is universal, deep-seated, and ultimately healthy, a need that is only heightened in gay men by their feeling so disconnected to the majority culture.

In essence, gay male couples straddle two cultures, mainstream society and the gay community. Some couples find the tension of living in two cultures difficult to endure. Like immigrants, they struggle with conflicting loyalties and values. We feel it is important that gay couples not lose their special qualities as gay men as they develop long-term relationships. Yet most of our ideas about long-term relationships come from the mainstream culture. For example, some gay men do not want to give up their nonmonogamy once they are in a long-term relationship because being sexually free is something of a badge of membership in the gay subculture and can serve as a protest against the mainstream culture. We believe it is extremely important to help the couple address the larger issues that may be influencing their behaviors, attitudes, and decisions about the rules of their relationship. If nonmonogamy is discovered ultimately to be about nonconformity just for the sake of it, or holding out for some personal autonomy to avoid a more authentic connectedness in the couple's relationship, the couple needs to struggle with this knowledge. Maybe anger at the mainstream culture can be expressed in other ways; maybe the one who wants more autonomy within the relationship can find another means to that end.

Gay men are in the process of creating and writing rules for their relationships. It is a time of exciting experimentation. Male couples have brought vitality into our clinical work, and we admire men's abilities to experiment in writing new scripts for themselves. Because gay couples, even after couple therapy, can often remain isolated and marginalized, we are working on a model of multiple couple groups for gay men to address those needs. We believe such a group might provide a context that supports male-to-male connectedness and that creates a peer environment for gay couples to learn from one another.

In this volume there are many important topics that we were not able to cover or have not covered in depth, including the impact of racism on gay men of color; substance abuse and the destabilizing impact of addiction on couples; the destructive influences of poverty; serodiscordant HIV couples; and the challenges for male couples in parenting and in growing old together. Although we see lesbian couples in our practices, neither of us felt we had sufficient expertise to write with innovation about their treatment.

In closing, every male couple we've ever met has a story. Therapists need to hear those stories and be respectful of them. At the same time, we feel it is crucial not to be hamstrung by the stories. Stories can constrain as well as liberate. Couples come to treatment ambivalent about change. They know that something needs to change, but following their old story lines, like traveling in worn grooves, is familiar, and thus comforting. In order for therapists to help a couple discover new grooves, the old ones have to be blocked. Challenge forces a couple to re-story itself, to write a new script, to cut some new grooves. Since many of the traditional scripts don't work so well (even for heterosexuals), couple therapy with gay men is a time for experimentation. Our therapy is unique in that we don't tell gay men which story is better for them. We disrupt them just enough so that they begin discovering their own new grooves and their own inherent resources. This part of doing the work is exciting. Once the couple starts experimenting with each other, the clinical work—and their relationship—takes off.

References

Ainsworth, M. D. S., Blehar, M. C., Waters, E., & Wall, S. (1978). *Patterns of attachment: A psychological study of the strange situation.* Hillsdale, NJ: Erlbaum.

Allen, J. P., & Land, D. (1999). Attachment in adolescence. In J. Cassidy & P. R. Shaver (Eds.), *Handbook of attachment: Theory, research, and clinical applications.* New York: Guilford Press.

Allport, G. (1958). *The nature of prejudice.* Garden City, NY: Doubleday.

American Psychiatric Association. (1994). *Diagnostic and statistical manual of mental disorders* (4th ed.). Washington, DC: Author.

Anderson, H., & Goolishian, H. A. (1988). Human systems as linguistic systems. *Family Process, 27,* 371–393.

Angyl, A. (1951). A theoretical model for personality studies. *Journal of Personality, 20,* 131–142.

Atkinson, L. (1997). Attachment and psychopathology: From laboratory to clinic. In L. Atkinson & K. J. Zucker (Eds.), *Attachment and psychopathology.* New York: Guilford Press.

Bailey, J. M., & Zucker, K. J. (1995). Childhood sex-typed behavior and sexual orientation: A conceptual analysis and quantitative review. *Developmental Psychology, 31,* 43–55.

Bakan, (1966). *The duality of human existence.* Chicago: Rand McNally.

Basow, S. A. (1992). *Gender: Stereotypes and roles* (3rd ed.). Pacific Grove, CA: Brooks/Cole.

Bateson, G. (1979). *Mind and nature.* New York: Dutton.

Bayer, R. (1987). *Homosexuality and American psychiatry: The politics of diagnosis* (2nd ed.). Princeton, NJ: Princeton University Press.

Bem, S. L. (1981). Gender schema theory: A cognitive account of sex typing. *Psychological Review, 88,* 354–364.

Bem, S. L. (1993). *The lenses of gender.* New Haven, CT: Yale University Press.

Blumstein, P., & Schwartz, P. (1983). *American couples: Money, work and sex.* New York: Morrow.

Bowen, M. (1966). The use of family theory in clinical practice. *Comprehensive Psychiatry, 7,* 345–374.

Bowen, M. (1978). *Family therapy in clinical practice.* New York: Aronson.

Bowlby, J. (1969/1982). *Attachment and loss: Vol. 1. Attachment.* New York: Basic Books.

Bowlby, J. (1973). *Attachment and loss: Vol. 2. Separation.* New York: Basic Books.

Bowlby, J. (1979). *The making and breaking of affectional bonds.* London: Tavistock.

Boyd-Franklin, N. (1989). *Black families in therapy: A multisystems approach.* New York: Guilford Press.

Boyd-Franklin, N. (1993). Race, class, and poverty. In F. Walsh (Ed.), *Normal family processes* (2nd ed.). New York: Guilford Press.

Brannon, R. (1976). The male sex role: Our culture's blueprint of manhood and what it's done for us lately. In D. David & R. Brannon (Eds.), *The 49-percent majority.* Reading, MA: Addison-Wesley.

Broido, E. M. (2000). Constructing identity: The nature and meaning of lesbian, gay, and bisexual identities. In R. M. Perez, K. A. DeBord, & K. J. Biescheke (Eds.), *Handbook of counseling and psychotherapy with lesbian, gay, and bisexual clients.* Washington, DC: American Psychological Association.

Carter, B., & McGoldrick, M. (Eds.). (1989). *The changing family life cycle: A framework for family therapy* (2nd ed.). Boston: Allyn & Bacon.

Carter, B., & McGoldrick, M. (Eds.). (1998). *The expanded family life cycle: Individual, family and social perspectives* (3rd ed.). Boston: Allyn & Bacon.

Cass, V. C. (1979). Homosexual identity formation: A theoretical model. *Journal of Homosexuality, 4,* 219–235.

Chodorow, N. (1978). *The reproduction of mothering: Psychoanalysis and the sociology of gender.* Berkeley, CA: University of California Press.

Colapinto, J. (1995). The dilution of family process in social services: Implications for treatment of neglectful families. *Family Process, 34 ,* 59–74.

Collins, N. L., & Read, S. J. (1990). Adult attachment, working models, and relationship quality in dating couples. *Journal of Personality and Social Psychology, 58,* 644–663.

Davison, G. C. (1991). Constructionism and morality in therapy for homosexuality. In J. C. Gonsiorek & J. D. Weinrich (Eds.), *Homosexuality: Research implications for public policy.* Newbury Park, CA: Sage.

Drescher, J. (1998). *Psychoanalytic therapy and the gay man.* Hillsdale, NJ: Analytic Press.

Duhl, E. J., Kantor, D., & Duhl, B. S. (1973). Learning space and action in family therapy: A primer in sculpture. In D. A. Block (Ed.), *Techniques of family psychotherapy.* New York: Grune & Stratton.

Erikson, E. H. (1950). *Childhood and society.* New York: Norton.

Feeney, J. A. (1999). Adult romantic attachment and couple relationships. In J. Cassidy & P. R. Shaver (Eds.), *Handbook of attachment: Theory, research, and clinical applications.* New York: Guilford Press.

Fogarty, T. F. (1979). The distancer and the pursuer. *The Family, 7,* 11–16.

Fonagy, P. (1999). Psychoanalytic theory from the viewpoint of attachment theory and research. In J. Cassidy & P. R. Shaver (Eds.), *Handbook of attachment: Theory, research, and clinical applications.* New York: Guilford Press.

Fosha, D. (2000). *The transforming power of affect: A model for accelerated change.* New York: Basic Books.

Genijovich, E. (1994). *The impossible blended family* [Videotape]. Boston: Family Studies, Inc.

Gerson, M.-J. (2001). A baby, maybe: Crossing the parenthood threshold. In S. McDaniel, D.-D. Lusterman, & C. L. Philpot (Eds.), *Casebook for integrating family therapy.* Washington, DC: American Psychological Association.

Gilligan, C. (1982). *In a different voice: Psychological theory and women's development.* Cambridge, MA: Harvard University Press.

Goffman, E. (1959). *The presentation of self in everyday life.* Garden City, NY: Doubleday.

Goffman, E. (1963). *Stigma: Notes on the management of spoiled identity.* Englewood Cliffs, NJ: Prentice-Hall.

Gonsiorek, J. C., & Rudolph, J. R. (1991). Homosexual identity: Coming out and other developmental events. In J. C. Gonsiorek & J. D. Weinrich (Eds.), *Homosexuality: Research implications for public policy.* Newbury Park, CA: Sage.

Gottman, J., Notarius, C., Gonso, J., & Markman, H. (1976). *A couple's guide to communication.* Champaign, IL: Research Press.

Green, R. (1987). *The "sissy boy syndrome" and the development of homosexuality.* New Haven, CT: Yale University Press.

Green, R.-J., Bettinger, M., & Zacks, E. (1996). Are lesbian couples fused and gay male couples disengaged? Questioning gender straightjackets. In J. Laird & R.-J. Green (Eds.), *Lesbians and gays in couples and families: A handbook for therapists.* San Francisco: Jossey-Bass.

Green, R.-J., & Mitchell, V. (2002). Gay and lesbian couples in therapy: Homophobia, relational ambiguity, and social support. In A. S. Gurman & N. S. Jacobson (Eds.), *Clinical handbook of couple therapy* (3rd ed.). New York: Guilford Press.

Greenan, D. (1987). *The hidden grievers* [Videotape]. New York: St. Vincent's Hospital and Medical Center.

Haley, J. (1987). *Problem solving therapy.* San Francisco: Jossey-Bass.

Hancock, K. A. (2000). Lesbian, gay and bisexual lives: Basic issues in psychotherapy training and practice. In B. Greene & G. L. Croom (Eds.), *Education, research, and practice in lesbian, gay, bisexual, and transgendered psychology: A resource manual*. Thousand Oaks, CA: Sage.

Hardy, K. (1993). War of the worlds. *Family Therapy Networker, 17*, 50–57.

Hazan, C., & Shaver, P. R. (1987). Romantic love conceptualized as an attachment process. *Journal of Personality and Social Psychology, 52*, 511–524.

Hazan, C., & Zeifman, D. (1999). Pair bonds as attachments: Evaluating the evidence. In J. Cassidy & P. R. Shaver (Eds.), *Handbook of attachment: Theory, research, and clinical applications*. New York: Guilford Press.

Holleran, A. (1978). *Dancer from the dance*. New York: Morrow.

Isay, R. A. (1989). *Being homosexual: Gay men and their development*. New York: Farrar Straus Giroux.

Johnson, S. M. (1999). Emotionally focused couple therapy: Straight to the heart. In J. M. Donovan (Ed.), *Short-term couple therapy*. New York: Guilford Press.

Johnson, S. M., Makinen, J. A., & Millikin, J. W. (2001). Attachment injuries in couple relationships: A new perspective on impasses in couples therapy. *Journal of Marital & Family Therapy, 27*, 145–156.

Johnson, T. W., & Keren, M. S. (1996). Creating and maintaining boundaries in male couples. In J. Laird & R.-J. Green (Eds.), *Lesbians and gays in couples and families: A handbook for therapists*. San Francisco: Jossey-Bass.

Kohlberg, L. A. (1966). A cognitive-developmental analysis of children's sex-role concepts and attitudes. In E. E. Maccoby (Ed.), *The development of sex differences*. Stanford, CA: Stanford University Press.

Kooden, H. (2000). *Golden men: The power of gay midlife*. New York: Avon Books.

Krestan, J. A., & Bepko, C. S. (1980). The problem of fusion in lesbian relationships. *Family Process, 19*, 277–289.

Kurdek, L. A. (1987). Sex-role self-schema and psychological adjustment in coupled homosexual and heterosexual men and women. *Sex Roles, 17*, 549–562.

Lusterman, D.-D. (1995). Treating marital infidelity. In R. Mikesell, D.-D. Lusterman, & S. McDaniel (Eds.), *Integrating family therapy: Handbook of family psychology and systems theory*. Washington, DC: American Psychological Association.

Martin, A. (1993). *The lesbian and gay parenting handbook: Creating and raising our families*. New York: HarperCollins.

Martin, A., & Tunnell, G. (1993). *Couples therapy with same-sex couples*. Workshop presented at the meeting of the Eastern Group Psychotherapy Society, New York.

McGoldrick, M., & Gerson, R. (1985). *Genograms in family assessment.* New York: Norton.

McWhirter, D. P., & Mattison, A. M. (1984). *The male couple: How relationships develop.* Englewood Cliffs, NJ: Prentice-Hall.

Minuchin, P., Colapinto, J., & Minuchin, S. (1998). *Working with families of the poor.* New York: Guilford Press.

Minuchin, S. (1974). *Families and family therapy.* Cambridge, MA: Harvard University Press.

Minuchin, S., & Fishman, C. (1981). *Family therapy techniques.* Cambridge, MA: Harvard University Press.

Minuchin, S., Lee, W. Y., & Simon, G. (1996). *Mastering family therapy: Journeys of growth and transformation.* New York: Wiley.

Minuchin, S., & Nichols, M. P. (1993). *Family healing: Tales of hope and renewal from family therapy.* New York: Free Press.

Mohr, J. J. (1999). Same-sex romantic attachment. In J. Cassidy & P. R. Shaver (Eds.), *Handbook of attachment: Theory, research, and clinical applications.* New York: Guilford Press.

Nichols, M. P. (1997). The art of enactment. *Family Therapy Networker, 21*(6), 23.

Nichols, M. P., & Fellenberg, S. (2000). The effective use of enactments in family therapy: A discovery-oriented process study. *Journal of Marital and Family Therapy, 26,* 143–152.

Nichols, M. P., & Minuchin, S. (1999). Short-term structural family therapy with couples. In J. M. Donovan (Ed.), *Short-term couple therapy.* New York: Guilford Press.

Nichols, M. P., & Schwartz, R. C. (1998). *Family therapy: concepts and methods.* Boston: Allyn & Bacon.

Nicolosi, J. (1991). *Reparative therapy of male homosexuality: A new clinical approach.* Northdale, NJ: Aronson.

Pillard, R. C. (1991). Masculinity and femininity in homosexual "inversion" revisited. In J. C. Gonsiorek & J. D. Weinrich (Eds.), *Homosexuality: Research implications for public policy.* Newbury Park, CA: Sage.

Pittman, F. (1987). *Turning points: Treating families in transition and crisis.* New York: Norton.

Rank, O. (1929). *The trauma of birth.* New York: Harcourt, Brace.

Rechy, J. (1977). *The sexual outlaw: A documentary.* New York: Dell.

Remafedi, G., French, S., Story, M., Resnick, M. D., & Blum, R. (1998). The relationship between suicide risk and sexual orientation: Results of a population-based survey. *American Journal of Public Health, 88,* 57–60.

Reynolds, A., & Hanjorgiris, W. F. (2000). Coming out: Lesbian, gay, and bisexual identity development. In R. M. Perez, K. A. DeBord, & K. J. Biescheke (Eds.), *Handbook of counseling and psychotherapy with lesbian, gay, and bisexual clients.* Washington, DC: American Psychological Association.

Rolland, J. S. (1987). Chronic illness and the life cycle: A conceptual framework. *Family Process, 26,* 203–221.

Rolland, J. S. (1994). *Helping families with chronic and life-threatening disorders.* New York: Basic Books.

Savin-Williams, R. C. (1998). *"And then I became gay": Young men's stories.* New York: Routledge.

Schnarch, D. (1997). *Passionate marriage: Sex, love and intimacy in emotionally committed relationships.* New York: Norton.

Shernoff, M. (1997). *Gay widowers: Life after the death of a partner.* New York: Harrington Park Press.

Shildo, A., Shroeder, M., & Drescher, J. (Eds.). (2002). *Sexual conversion therapy: Ethical, clinical, and research perspectives.* New York: Haworth.

Siegel, S., & Walker, G. (1999). Connections: Conversations between a gay therapist and a straight therapist. In J. Laird & R.-J. Green (Eds.), *Lesbians and gays in couples and families: A handbook for therapists.* San Francisco: Jossey-Bass.

Sullivan, A. (1996, November 10). When plagues end. *New York Times Magazine* pp. 52–62, 76–77, 84.

Thompson, R. A. (1999). Early attachment and later development. In J. Cassidy & P. R. Shaver (Eds.), *Handbook of attachment: Theory, research, and clinical applications.* New York: Guilford Press.

Tunnell, G. (1991). Complications in group psychotherapy with AIDS patients. *International Journal of Group Psychotherapy, 41,* 481–498.

Warner, M. (1999). *The trouble with normal: Sex, politics, and the ethics of queer life.* Cambridge, MA: Harvard University Press.

Werner, P. D., Green, R.-J., Greenberg, J., Browne, T. L., & McKenna, T. E. (2001). Beyond enmeshment: Evidence for the independence of intrusiveness and closeness-caregiving in married couples. *Journal of Marital and Family Therapy, 27,* 459–471.

Westin, K. (1991). *Families we choose: Lesbians, gays, kinship.* New York: Columbia University Press.

Winnicott, D. W. (1965). *The maturational process and the facilitating environment.* New York: International Universities Press.

Wright, F. (1994). Men, shame and group psychotherapy. *Group, 18,* 212–224.

Index

"f" indicates a figure; "n" indicates a note

214 Index

V

Videotaping
  benefits of, 130–136
  introducing to clients, 83
  joining phase of treatment, 52–53f
  monitoring interventions, 153
  separation from the content, 170

Vulnerability
  addressing in therapy, 16
  expressing within relationships, 13–15

W

Waiting room literature, 81
"We-ness," language of, 65, 179, 190